TOP TRAILS™

Sequoia and Kings Canyon National Parks

MUST-DO HIKES FOR EVERYONE

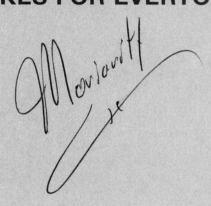

Written by

Mike White

WILDERNESS PRESS ... *on the trail since 1967*

Top Trails Sequoia and Kings Canyon National Parks: Must-Do Hikes for Everyone

1st EDITION 2009
  3rd printing 2013

Copyright © 2009 by Mike White

All photos copyright © 2009 by Mike White, except where noted
Maps: Mike White
Cover design: Frances Baca Design and Lisa Pletka
Interior design: Frances Baca Design
Book production: Larry B. Van Dyke and Lisa Pletka
Book editors: Laura Shauger and Joe Walowski

ISBN 978-0-89997-486-6

Manufactured in the United States of America

Published by: **Wilderness Press**
               Keen Communication
               PO Box 43673
               Birmingham, AL 35243
               (800) 443-7227; FAX (205) 326-1012
               info@wildernesspress.com
               www.wildernesspress.com
Visit our website for a complete listing of our books and for ordering information.
Distributed by Publishers Group West

Cover photos: Long Lake, John Muir Wilderness (Trail 29) copyright © 2009
              by Londie G. Padelsky/Larry Ulrich Stock Photography;
              giant sequoias (inset) copyright © 2009 by Roslyn Bullas

The Top Trails™ Series

Wilderness Press

When Wilderness Press published *Sierra North* in 1967, no other trail guide like it existed for the Sierra backcountry. The first print run sold out in less than two months and its success heralded the beginning of Wilderness Press. Since we were founded more than 40 years ago, we have expanded our territories to cover California, Alaska, Hawaii, the U.S. Southwest, the Pacific Northwest, the Midwest, the Southeast, New England, Canada, and Baja California.

Wilderness Press continues to publish comprehensive, accurate, and readable outdoor books. Hikers, backpackers, kayakers, skiers, snowshoers, climbers, cyclists, and trail runners rely on Wilderness Press for accurate outdoor adventure information.

Top Trails

In its Top Trails guides, Wilderness Press has paid special attention to organization so that you can find the perfect hike each and every time. Whether you're looking for a steep trail to test yourself on or a walk in the park, a romantic waterfall or a city view, Top Trails will lead you there.

Each Top Trails guide contains trails for everyone. The trails selected provide a sampling of the best that the region has to offer. These are the "must-do" hikes, walks, runs, and bike rides, with every feature of the area represented.

Every book in the Top Trails series offers:

- The Wilderness Press commitment to accuracy and reliability
- Ratings and rankings for each trail
- Distances and approximate times
- Easy-to-follow trail notes
- Maps and permit information

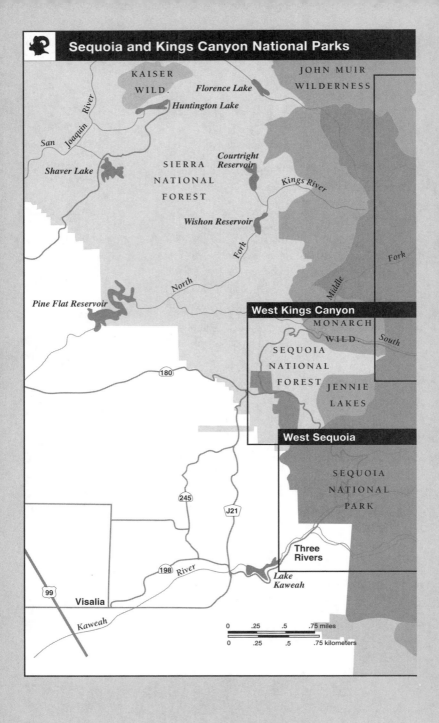

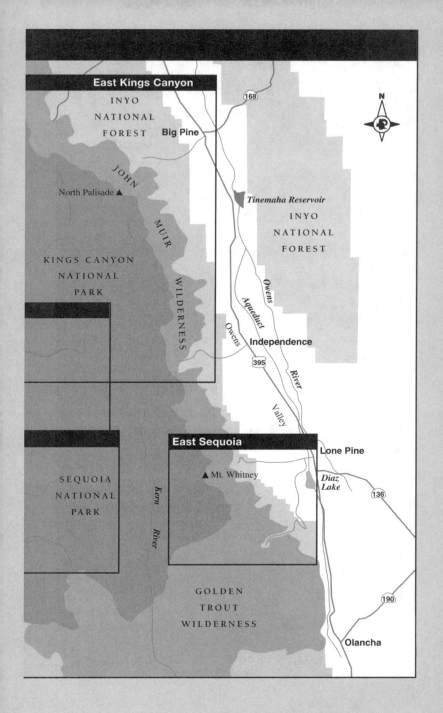

Sequoia and Kings Canyon Trails

TRAIL NUMBER AND NAME	Page	Difficulty -12345+	Length in Miles	Type	Dayhiking	Backpacking	Running	Horseback Riding	Dogs Allowed
1. West Sequoia									
1 Putnam and Snowslide Canyons	37	3	6.8	Out & Back	Dayhiking		Running	Horses	
2 Paradise Peak	41	4	9.6	Out & Back	Dayhiking		Running	Horses	
3 Eagle Lake	47	4	6.5	Out & Back	Dayhiking	Backpacking	Running	Horses	
4 Monarch Lakes	53	4	6.5	Out & Back	Dayhiking	Backpacking	Running	Horses	
5 Potwisha Pictographs Loop	59	1	0.5	Loop	Dayhiking				
6 Marble Falls	63	3	6.8	Out & Back	Dayhiking				
7 Crescent and Log Meadows Loop	67	2	2.4	Loop	Dayhiking				
8 Congress Trail	73	2	3.1	Loop	Dayhiking				
9 Circle Meadow Loop	79	2	5.8	Loop	Dayhiking				
10 Alta Peak	85	5	13.4	Out & Back	Dayhiking	Backpacking		Horses	
11 Heather, Aster, Emerald, and Pear Lakes	91	4	11.5	Out & Back	Dayhiking	Backpacking		Horses	
12 Tokopah Falls	99	2	4.1	Out & Back	Dayhiking			Horses	
13 Little Baldy	103	3	3.5	Out & Back	Dayhiking				
14 Muir Grove	107	3	4.2	Out & Back	Dayhiking				
2. West Kings Canyon									
15 Big Baldy	123	3	4.4	Out & Back	Dayhiking		Running		
16 Redwood Mountain Grove	127	3	7.25, 6.6	Loop	Dayhiking	Backpacking	Running		
17 Mitchell Peak	137	4	6.0	Out & Back	Dayhiking		Running		
18 Sunset Loop Trail	141	3	6.4	Loop	Dayhiking		Running		
19 General Grant Tree Trail	149	1	0.5	Loop	Dayhiking				
20 Panoramic Point and Park Ridge Lookout	153	3	5.6	Loop	Dayhiking		Running		
21 Boole Tree	157	2	4.5	Loop	Dayhiking				
22 Lookout Peak	161	4	10.0	Out & Back	Dayhiking		Running		
23 Roaring River Falls	165	1	0.5	Out & Back	Dayhiking				
24 Zumwalt Meadow Nature Trail	169	1	1.5	Loop	Dayhiking				
25 Kanawyer Loop Trail	173	2	4.7	Loop	Dayhiking		Running	Horses	

TYPE

- Loop
- Out & Back

DIFFICULTY
-12345+
less more

USES & ACCESS

- Dayhiking
- Backpacking
- Running
- Horses
- Dogs Allowed
- Handicapped Access
- Child Friendly

TERRAIN

- Canyon
- Mountain
- Summit
- Lake
- River or Stream
- Waterfall

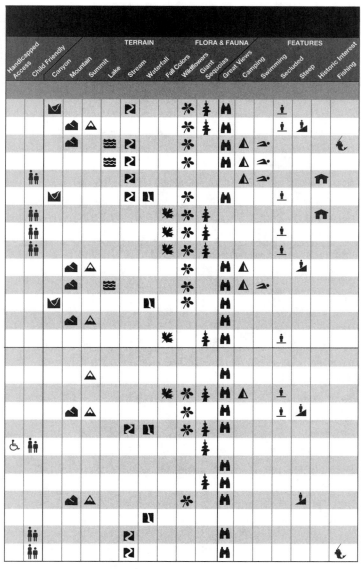

Handicapped Access	Child Friendly	TERRAIN						FLORA & FAUNA			FEATURES						
		Canyon	Mountain	Summit	Lake	Stream	Waterfall	Fall Colors	Wildflowers	Giant Sequoias	Great Views	Camping	Swimming	Secluded	Steep	Historic Interest	Fishing
		●				●			●	●	●			●			
			●	●					●	●	●			●	●		
			●		●	●			●		●	●	●				●
			●		●	●			●		●	●	●				
	●					●						●	●			●	
		●				●	●		●		●			●			
	●							●	●	●						●	
	●							●	●	●				●			
	●							●	●	●				●			
			●	●					●		●	●			●		
			●		●				●		●	●	●				
		●					●		●		●						
			●	●							●						
								●		●	●			●			
				●							●						
								●	●	●	●	●		●			
			●	●					●		●			●	●		
						●	●		●	●	●						
●	●									●							
											●						
										●	●						
			●	●					●		●				●		
							●										
	●					●					●						
	●					●					●						●

FLORA & FAUNA

🍁 Fall Colors
❀ Wildflowers
🌲 Giant Sequoias

FEATURES

Great Views
Camping
Swimming
Secluded
Steep
Historic Interest
Fishing

Sequoia and Kings Canyon Trails

Trail Number and Name	Page	Difficulty -1 2 3 4 5+	Length in Miles	Type	Dayhiking	Backpacking	Running	Horseback Riding	Dogs Allowed
26 Mist Falls	177	3	7.8	Out & Back	Dayhiking		Running	Horseback Riding	
27 Hotel and Lewis Creeks Loop	181	4	6.4	Loop	Dayhiking		Running	Horseback Riding	

3. Golden Trout Wilderness, John Muir Wilderness, and East Sequoia

Trail Number and Name	Page	Difficulty	Length in Miles	Type	Dayhiking	Backpacking	Running	Horseback Riding	Dogs Allowed
28 Chicken Spring Lake	197	3	8.2	Out & Back	Dayhiking	Backpacking	Running	Horseback Riding	
29 South Fork, Cirque, Long, and High Lakes	201	3	13.0	Out & Back	Dayhiking	Backpacking	Running	Horseback Riding	Dogs Allowed
30 Soldier Lakes	207	4	22.0	Out & Back	Dayhiking	Backpacking	Running	Horseback Riding	
31 Cottonwood Lakes	215	3	11.8	Out & Back	Dayhiking	Backpacking	Running	Horseback Riding	Dogs Allowed
32 Meysan Trail	221	4	9	Out & Back	Dayhiking	Backpacking	Running		
33 Mount Whitney	225	5	22.0	Out & Back	Dayhiking	Backpacking	Running		

4. John Muir Wilderness and East Kings Canyon

Trail Number and Name	Page	Difficulty	Length in Miles	Type	Dayhiking	Backpacking	Running	Horseback Riding	Dogs Allowed
34 Robinson Lake	249	3	3.0	Out & Back	Dayhiking	Backpacking	Running		Dogs Allowed
35 Kearsarge and Bullfrog Lakes	253	4	14.2	Out & Back	Dayhiking	Backpacking	Running	Horseback Riding	
36 Charlotte Lake	261	4	16.5	Out & Back	Dayhiking	Backpacking	Running	Horseback Riding	
37 Golden Trout Lakes	267	4	4.4	Out & Back	Dayhiking	Backpacking	Running	Horseback Riding	Dogs Allowed
38 Red Lake	273	5	9.0	Out & Back	Dayhiking	Backpacking	Running		Dogs Allowed
39 Birch Lake	279	4	11.0	Out & Back	Dayhiking	Backpacking	Running		Dogs Allowed
40 Brainerd Lake	283	4	10.0	Out & Back	Dayhiking	Backpacking	Running	Horseback Riding	Dogs Allowed
41 Big Pine Lakes	289	4	11.4	Loop	Dayhiking	Backpacking	Running	Horseback Riding	Dogs Allowed
42 Long, Saddlerock, and Bishop Lakes	301	3	8.6	Out & Back	Dayhiking	Backpacking	Running	Horseback Riding	Dogs Allowed
43 Dusy Basin	307	4	15.2	Out & Back	Dayhiking	Backpacking	Running		
44 Chocolate Lakes Loop	315	3	7.2	Loop	Dayhiking	Backpacking	Running	Horseback Riding	Dogs Allowed
45 Treasure Lakes	321	3	7.6	Out & Back	Dayhiking	Backpacking	Running	Horseback Riding	Dogs Allowed
46 Tyee Lakes	327	3	6.5	Out & Back	Dayhiking	Backpacking	Running	Horseback Riding	Dogs Allowed
47 Sabrina Basin	333	3	13.6	Out & Back	Dayhiking	Backpacking	Running	Horseback Riding	Dogs Allowed
48 George Lake	341	3	6.6	Out & Back	Dayhiking	Backpacking	Running	Horseback Riding	Dogs Allowed
49 Lamarck Lakes	345	4	5.4	Out & Back	Dayhiking	Backpacking	Running	Horseback Riding	Dogs Allowed
50 Piute Pass Trail to Humphreys Basin	351	4	14.4	Out & Back	Dayhiking	Backpacking	Running	Horseback Riding	Dogs Allowed

TYPE
- ⟳ Loop
- ↗ Out & Back
- DIFFICULTY
  - 1 2 3 4 5 +
  - less   more

USES & ACCESS
- Dayhiking
- Backpacking
- Running
- Horseback Riding
- Dogs Allowed
- Handicapped Access
- Child Friendly

TERRAIN
- Canyon
- Mountain
- Summit
- Lake
- River or Stream
- Waterfall

Handicapped Access	Child Friendly	Canyon	Mountain	Summit	Lake	Stream	Waterfall	Fall Colors	Wildflowers	Giant Sequoias	Great Views	Camping	Swimming	Secluded	Steep	Historic Interest	Fishing
👫	✓					✓	✓										✓
	✓					✓			✓		✓						
		✓			✓						✓	✓	✓				
		✓			✓							✓	✓				
	✓	✓			✓	✓			✓		✓	✓	✓				
		✓			✓							✓	✓				✓
	✓	✓			✓				✓			✓	✓		✓		
	✓	✓		✓					✓		✓	✓			✓		
		✓			✓	✓						✓	✓		✓		
		✓			✓				✓		✓	✓	✓				✓
		✓			✓				✓		✓	✓	✓				✓
		✓			✓				✓			✓	✓				✓
		✓			✓				✓			✓	✓	✓	✓		✓
		✓			✓				✓			✓	✓	✓			✓
		✓			✓				✓		✓	✓	✓				✓
		✓			✓				✓		✓	✓	✓			✓	✓
		✓			✓				✓		✓	✓	✓				✓
		✓			✓				✓			✓	✓				✓
		✓			✓				✓			✓	✓				✓
		✓			✓				✓			✓	✓				✓
		✓			✓				✓			✓	✓				✓
		✓			✓				✓			✓	✓				
		✓			✓				✓			✓	✓				✓
		✓			✓				✓			✓	✓				✓

FLORA & FAUNA
🍁 Fall Colors
❀ Wildflowers
🌲 Giant Sequoias

FEATURES
🔭 Great Views
⛺ Camping
🏊 Swimming
🧍 Secluded
⬇ Steep
🏠 Historic Interest
🎣 Fishing

Contents

CHAPTER 3

Golden Trout Wilderness, John Muir Wilderness, and East Sequoia 187

CHAPTER 4

John Muir Wilderness and East Kings Canyon 235

Using Top Trails™

Organization of Top Trails

Top Trails is designed to make identifying the perfect trail easy and enjoyable, and to make every outing a success and a pleasure. With this book you'll find it's a snap to find the right trail, whether you're planning a major hike or just a sociable stroll with friends.

The Region

Top Trails begins with the **Sequoia and Kings Canyon National Parks Map** (pages iv-v), displaying the entire region covered by the guide and providing a geographic overview. The map is clearly marked to show which area is covered by each chapter.

After the regional map comes the **Sequoia and Kings Canyon National Park Trails Table** (pages vi-ix), which lists every trail covered in the guide,

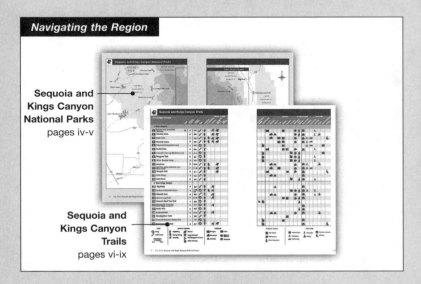

Navigating the Region

Sequoia and Kings Canyon National Parks
pages iv-v

Sequoia and Kings Canyon Trails
pages vi-ix

along with attributes for each trail. A quick reading of the regional map and the trails table will give you a good overview of the entire region covered by the book.

The Areas

The region covered in each book is divided into areas, with each chapter corresponding to one area in the region.

Each area chapter starts with information to help you choose and enjoy a trail every time out. Use the table of contents or the regional map to identify an area of interest, then turn to the area chapter to find the following:

- An overview of the area, including park and permit information
- An area map with all trails clearly marked
- A trail feature table providing trail-by-trail details
- Trail summaries written in a lively, accessible style

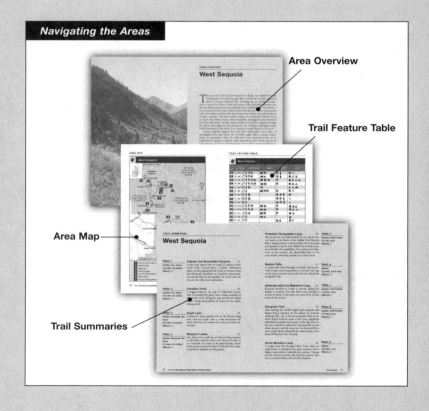

Navigating the Areas

Area Overview

Trail Feature Table

Area Map

Trail Summaries

The Trails

The basic building block of each Top Trails guide is the trail entry. Each one is arranged to make finding and following the trail as simple as possible, with all pertinent information presented in this easy-to-follow format:

- A trail map
- Trail descriptors covering difficulty, length, and other essential data
- A written trail description
- Trail milestones providing easy-to-follow, turn-by-turn trail directions

Some trail descriptions offer additional information:

- An elevation profile
- Trail options
- Trail highlights

In the margins of the trail entries, keep your eyes open for graphic icons that signal passages in the text.

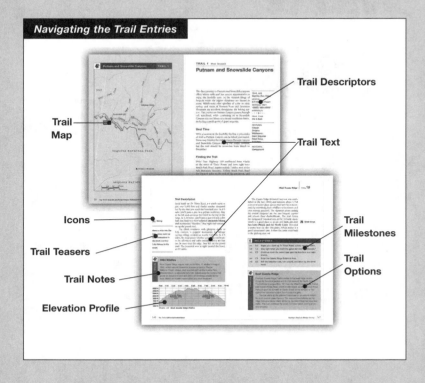

Choosing a Trail

Top Trails provides several different ways of choosing a trail, all presented in easy-to-read tables, charts, and maps.

Location

If you know in general where you want to go, Top Trails makes it easy to find the right trail in the right place. Each chapter begins with a large-scale map showing the starting point of every trail in that area.

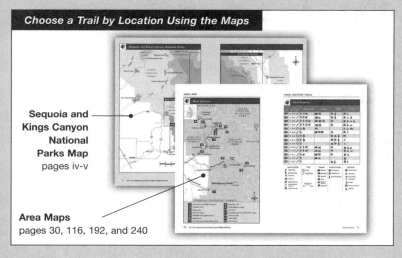

Choose a Trail by Location Using the Maps

Sequoia and Kings Canyon National Parks Map pages iv-v

Area Maps pages 30, 116, 192, and 240

Features

This guide describes the top trails of the Sequoia and Kings Canyon National Park region. Each trail has been chosen because it offers one or more features that make it interesting. Using the trail descriptors, summaries, and tables, you can quickly examine all the trails for the features they offer, or seek a particular feature among the list of trails.

Season and Condition

Time of year and current conditions can be important factors in selecting the best trail. For example, an exposed grassland trail may be a riot of color in early spring, but an oven-baked taste of hell in midsummer. Wherever relevant, Top Trails identifies the best and worst conditions for the trails you plan to hike.

Difficulty

Each trail has an overall difficulty rating on a scale of 1 to 5, which takes into consideration length, elevation change, exposure, trail quality, and more, to create one (admittedly subjective) rating.

The ratings assume you are an able-bodied adult in reasonably good shape using the trail for hiking. The ratings also assume normal weather conditions—clear and dry.

Readers should make an honest assessment of their own abilities and adjust time estimates accordingly. Also, rain, snow, heat, and poor visibility can all affect the pace on even the easiest of trails.

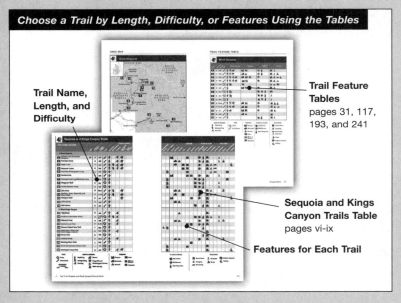

Choose a Trail by Length, Difficulty, or Features Using the Tables

Trail Name, Length, and Difficulty

Trail Feature Tables
pages 31, 117, 193, and 241

Sequoia and Kings Canyon Trails Table
pages vi–ix

Features for Each Trail

Vertical Feet

This important measurement is often underestimated by hikers and bikers when gauging the difficulty of a trail. The Top Trails measurement accounts for all elevation change, not simply the difference between the highest and lowest points, so that rolling terrain with lots of ups and downs, will be identifiable.

The calculation of vertical feet in the Top Trails series is accomplished by a combination of trail measurement and computer-aided estimation. For routes that begin and end at the same spot—i.e., loop or out and back—the vertical gain exactly matches the vertical descent. With a point-to-point route, the vertical gain and loss will most likely differ, and both figures will be provided in the text.

For one-way trips, the elevation gain is listed first, and the loss figure follows. For loops or out-and-back trips, the elevation figures are the total gain and loss for the entire trip. The last number is the total gain plus loss for the entire trip.

Finally, some trail entries in the Top Trails series have an elevation profile, an easy means for visualizing the topography of the route. These profiles graphically depict the elevation throughout the length of the trail.

 Top Trails Difficulty Ratings

1   A short trail, generally level, which can be completed in one hour or less.

2   A route of 1 to 3 miles, with some up and down, which can be completed in one to two hours.

3   A longer route, up to 5 miles, with uphill and/or downhill sections.

4   A long or steep route, perhaps more than 5 miles, or with climbs of more than 1000 vertical feet.

5   The most severe route, both long and steep, more than 5 miles long, with climbs of more than 1000 vertical feet.

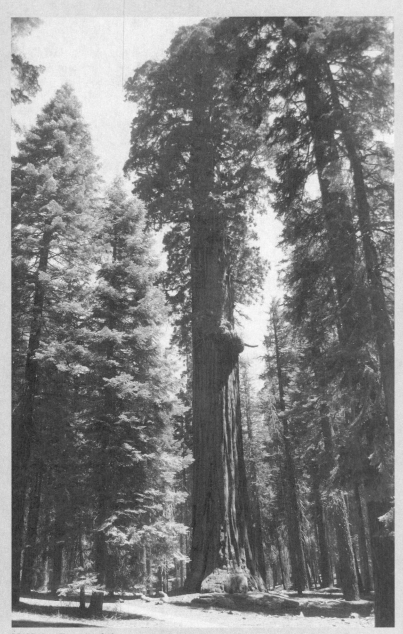

McKinley Tree (*Trail 8*)

Introduction to Sequoia and Kings Canyon National Parks

Somewhat less well known by tourists than neighboring Yosemite, Sequoia and Kings Canyon is nonetheless revered by outdoor enthusiasts from around the globe as containing some of the most coveted backcountry in the world. A large portion of the distinguished John Muir Trail and all of the High Sierra Trail lies within the parks, as does the Lower 48's highest mountain, Mt. Whitney, and the world's largest tree, General Sherman. As one of North America's deepest gorges, Kings Canyon is another important feature of the region that draws a host of sightseers, campers, hikers, backpackers, equestrians, and anglers. Protecting a large area of prime Sierra Nevada topography, Sequoia and Kings Canyon leaves a lasting impression on all who are fortunate enough to experience this marvelous national treasure.

The spectacular terrain within the current configuration of Sequoia and Kings Canyon was not fully set aside as national parkland until fairly recently. Although the first legislation to protect any of these lands was approved as far back as 1880, when Theodore Wagner, then U.S. Surveyor General for California, suspended 4 square miles of Grant Grove from application for land claims. The next 85 years saw various threats to the preservation of the Sequoia and Kings Canyon area from water, timber, mining, and development interests. After decades of advocacy from private citizens and government servants alike, including such notables as John Muir himself, the stunning landscape we know today was mostly set aside as Sequoia and Kings Canyon national parks in 1965. However, national park status failed to confer complete protection to all these lands until 1978 when, after the Sierra Club successfully defeated the Walt Disney Company's bid to develop a destination ski resort, the Mineral King area was added to the parklands.

Whirlwind Tour

Although this book is primarily a hiking guide, if you plan to visit the parks for just one day, you'll hardly have time to get out of your vehicle. Higher gas prices have greatly limited the appetite of the masses for the old-fashioned Sunday drive but, if you don't mind the expense, you can sample some of the wonders of Sequoia and Kings Canyon on a one-day auto tour.

From the town of Three Rivers on State Highway 198, with a full tank of gas, drive into Sequoia National Park via the Ash Mountain Entrance and the Generals Highway to the **Foothills Visitors Center**, where you can get acclimated to the park and obtain information about roads and facilities.

Continue on the Generals Highway along Middle Fork Kaweah River until the road eventually makes a stiff, winding climb out of the canyon and up to the Giant Forest. Park your vehicle in the large lot across from the **Giant Forest Museum** and take a tour of the museum before boarding the free shuttle bus to Moro Rock. Hike the short, steep, quarter-mile-long path to the top of **Moro Rock** for the incredible view. Afterward, ride the shuttle back to Giant Forest, transfer to the free shuttle to the Sherman Tree bus stop and walk the very short loop around the **General Sherman Tree**. From there, ride the shuttle bus back to the Giant Forest and pick up your vehicle.

Continue on Generals Highway away from the Giant Forest. By now you should be ready for lunch, which you can pro- cure either at the Watchtower Deli or Harrison BBQ & Grill in **Lodgepole**, or the dining room at **Wuksachi Village**. If you prefer to picnic, pack a basket beforehand and enjoy lunch at **Halstead picnic area**.

Geography and Topography

The Sequoia-Kings Canyon region is blessed with some of the most magnificent scenery in North America, including one of the deepest canyons, 8000-foot deep Kings Canyon, and the tallest mountain in the Lower 48, Mt. Whitney at 14,494 feet. The Kern, San Joaquin, Kaweah, and Kings rivers all begin here, flowing westward through dramatic canyons on their way to the plain of the agriculturally verdant San Joaquin Valley below. Along with Mt. Whitney, the High Sierra offers up numerous peaks topping out at 12,000 to 14,000 feet. The range rises gradually out of the San Joaquin Valley, first through the characteristic oak woodland of the foothills and then

After lunch, follow Generals Highway past Lost Grove and proceed through Giant Sequoia National Monument to Kings Canyon National Park. At the intersection of Highway 180, veer right and drive a short distance to **Grant Grove Village**. Just past the visitors center, turn right and follow Panoramic Point Road 2.3 miles to the parking area at the end of the road. Take the quarter-mile path to the viewpoint for a superb vista of the Great Western Divide and Sierra Crest from **Panorama Point**. Afterward, return to Highway 180.

Bound ultimately for the deep cleft of Kings Canyon, proceed out of the park on Highway 180, cresting the road's high point at Cherry Gap, before starting the long descent into the canyon. Stop at **Boyden Cavern** for the 45-minute, guided tour for which you must pay a fee.

From the cavern, drive Highway 180 along the South Fork Kings River back into Kings Canyon National Park and up Kings Canyon past Cedar Grove to the turnout for **Roaring River Falls**. Walk the very short paved path to the falls viewpoint and return to the parking area. From there, continue up the highway to the **Zumwalt Meadow Nature Trail** and take the 1.5-mile, nearly level path around the meadow, which offers good views of the river from a bridge and the vertical, Yosemite-like canyon walls. Back at the car, drive up the canyon to Roads End and then loop back to **Cedar Grove Village**. At Cedar Grove, you can grab a burger at the restaurant, or pick up deli items from the market and enjoy a picnic on the grounds nearby.

Conclude your long day by driving Highway 180 back to Grant Grove and then out of the park toward Fresno.

a grand belt of forest on the way to the towering, glacial sculpted alpine crest of granite peaks along the spine of the High Sierra. From there, the landscape tumbles steeply in dramatic fashion toward the basin of the Owens Valley. The vertical relief of this eastern escarpment as measured from the top of Mt. Whitney to the town of Lone Pine at the mountain's base is a staggering 10,760 feet (all in a mere 13 air miles) and is the greatest relief in the continental U.S.

The two parks, managed by the National Park Service as one unit, have a combined area of 862,103 acres, more than 90 percent of which is managed as wilderness. With more than 800 miles of trail, the parks are a virtual nirvana for hikers, backpackers, and equestrians. Adding in the acreage and trail mileage of the neighboring John Muir, Golden Trout, Jennie Lakes,

Monarch, and Dinkey Lakes wilderness areas, the region is one of the largest roadless areas in the West. Fortunate visitors will find towering granite peaks, picturesque mountain lakes, dramatic glacier-carved canyons with clear running streams and cascading waterfalls, lush meadows filled with colorful wildflowers, and dense forests of magnificent trees. Pockets of those forests include the most magnificent tree of all, the giant sequoia, touted as the largest living species of tree in the world. While having some areas of focused visitation, namely Giant Forest, Lodgepole, Grant Grove, and Cedar Grove, the two parks escape the concentration of tourists so common to Yosemite National Park to the north.

Geology

Most of the land within the greater Sequoia-Kings Canyon region is granitic. These light-colored, salt-and-pepper speckled, coarse-grained rocks include granite, granodiorite, and tonalite (formerly referred to as quartz diorite). A large mass of granitic rock, 300 miles long and at points more than 50 miles wide, which geologists call the Sierra Nevada Batholith, was uplifted and exposed over a long period of geologic time to transform into the characteristic granite landscape known today as the Sierra Nevada. In addition to the overwhelming amount of granite, a small percentage of the rock in the Sierra is metamorphic. Darker in color and variegated in appearance, these metamorphic rocks are older than the granitic rocks. Remnants of these older rocks are scattered across the Sequoia-Kings Canyon region. An even smaller amount of the area's composition includes volcanic rock, although within the park's boundaries volcanic rock is almost nonexistent. The most extensive area of volcanic rock in the region is located just east of Kings Canyon National Park in the Big Pine Volcanic Field, visible by motorists from U.S. Highway 395.

The Sequoia-Kings Canyon region is home to some of the most impressive canyons in North America. Both stream erosion and glaciation have greatly influenced these canyons. At lower elevations, the power of water is clearly evident in the carving of V-shaped canyons. In the higher elevations, classic U-shaped canyons bear the evidence of glacial formation.

Speculation about the role of glaciers in the sculpting of the Sierra Nevada dates back to John Muir's day. Whatever their importance in the past, glaciers in today's Sierra Nevada are nearly insignificant in size and depth and will certainly be even more so in the future thanks to global warming. Despite their lack of volume, the small number of remaining glaciers found at high elevations on shady north- and east-facing slopes add touches of alpine beauty to the rocky summits and dramatic faces of the High Sierra.

Flora and Fauna

Since the greater Sequoia-Kings Canyon region encompasses elevations from 2000 to over 14,000 feet, you can expect to see a diverse cross section of plant and animal life. Heading from west to east, the first zone encountered is the Sierra **foothills**, a low-elevation area that begins just east of the San Joaquin Valley and extends upward to around 4500 to 5000 feet. Characterized by a Mediterranean climate, the foothills include areas of grasslands, oak woodland, and chaparral. Poison oak is common here and you should be equipped to identify and avoid this three-leaved plant. A wide range of critters call the foothills home, including a variety of amphibians and reptiles. Although the western rattlesnake lives in the foothills, you're not likely to see one on the trail. Common small to medium mammals include rabbits, squirrels, rats, mice, raccoons, skunks, and coyotes. Mule deer and the seldom-seen bobcat and mountain lion make up the larger mammals in this zone. Numerous birds reside in the foothills—far too many to list even the most common species. Raptors include the red-tailed hawk, golden eagle, American kestrel, and great horned owl.

The next zone on your eastward journey through the Sierra Nevada is the **montane forest**. Ranging in elevation from 4500 to 7000 feet, the area is composed of both conifers, such as ponderosa pine, Jeffrey pine, white

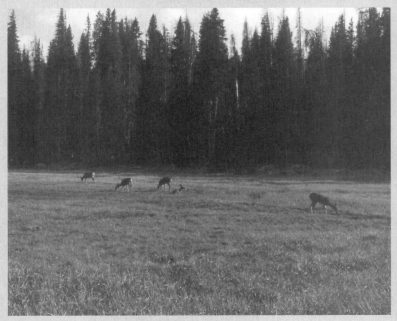

Deer grazing in Hockett Meadow

fir, sugar pine, and incense cedar, and deciduous trees, such as black oak and dogwood. Along streams, the montane forest supports a diverse array of riparian foliage. Amphibians and reptiles are common here, as they are in the foothills. In addition to many of the mammals of the foothill zone, the montane forest is home to black bears, porcupines, and weasels. A wide assortment of birds includes songbirds, woodpeckers, and raptors.

In areas of moist soil between 4500 and 8400 feet, 75 groves of **giant sequoias** are found sprinkled along the west side of the Sierra Nevada, the only place in the world to witness these monarchs of the forest. The highest concentration of giant sequoias is found within Sequoia and Kings Canyon national parks. The groves are not pure stands, but include white fir, incense cedar, sugar pine, and dogwood. Mature giant sequoias can reach heights of 150 to 300 feet and widths of 5 to 30 feet. Although quite massive in height and width, giant sequoias have very shallow root systems. The most common cause of death is not disease, infestation, or fire (thanks to their thick bark) but simply toppling over. Animal life in the giant sequoia groves is similar to that in the montane forest.

Moving up in elevation, between 7000 and 9000 feet is the **red fir forest**, where the namesake tree is frequently the sole species of this climax forest. Pure stands of red fir can be so dense that competitors and understory plants cannot survive if they aren't shade-tolerant. Where red firs are less dense, lodgepole pines, western white pines, Jeffrey pines, western junipers, and quaking aspens may join the forest. In addition, white fir may intermingle with red fir along the lower edge of this zone. The red fir zone receives the highest amounts of precipitation in the Sierra, which falls mainly as snow during the winter. Animals must adapt to the harsher conditions in this zone, which consequently limits the number of amphibians and reptiles. However, a wide variety of mammals seem to flourish here, including mice, gophers, voles, shrews, pikas, chipmunks, squirrels, rabbits, marmots, foxes, porcupines, coyotes, weasels, wolverines, badgers,

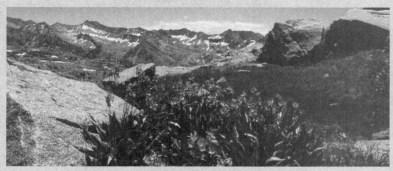

Wildflowers near Thunderbolt Pass, *Knapsack Pass cross-country*

pine martens, mule deer, and black bears. A diverse number of birds live in the red fir forest; some of the more interesting birds include blue grouse, dipper, and mountain bluebird.

Between 8000 and 11,000 feet is the **lodgepole pine forest**. This two-needled pine is one of the most common trees of the American West. Commonly found in pure stands, lodgepoles do intermix in areas with western white pines and, in the higher elevations, whitebark pines. Where abundant groundwater is present, quaking aspens also may be found with lodgepoles. Animal life is similar to that in the red fir forest.

Occurring between 9500 and 12,000 feet, the **subalpine zone** straddles the Sierra Crest and bridges the gap between the mighty forests of the lower altitudes and the much more austere realm above timberline. The most dominant conifer is the foxtail pine, a five-needled pine with pendulous branches, similar in appearance to the bristlecone pine. The most common associate is the whitebark pine, a multitrunked tree that grows in the harsh conditions just below timberline, oftentimes in the form of a windblown shrub. Mountain lakes, craggy peaks, and granite slabs and boulders fill breaks in the forest, as well as numerous meadows carpeted with lush grasses, sedges, and wildflowers. Animal life is similar to that in the red fir forest.

The **alpine zone** carpets the uppermost elevations of the High Sierra, where the growing season is measured in weeks rather than months. Lower temperatures and cloudier skies allow snow patches to linger here throughout the summer, despite the fact that the alpine zone actually receives less precipitation than zones below. With altitudes above 12,000 feet, frost can occur at any point in the summer, and cool temperatures and nearly constant winds combine with the lack of moisture to produce desertlike conditions. The generally poor, granitic soil further limits the ability of plant species to adapt to this environment. Most plants in the alpine zone are perennial and have developed a low-growing, compact, and drought-tolerant form, which allows them to avoid the strongest winds, grow closer to the warmth of the soil, and survive on small amounts of moisture.

The alpine zone can be subdivided into two classifications: alpine meadow and alpine rock. Alpine meadows are common where a sufficient layer of soil is present. Composed principally of sedges and a limited number of grasses, colorful wildflowers put on a showy display in alpine meadows during the brief summer. Unlike the broad swaths of foliage in alpine meadows, small patches of vegetation make up the plant life in the alpine rock community, where open gravel flats produce a smattering of alpine plants and protected areas in boulder fields host a wide array of wildflowers.

Aside from insects and invertebrates, few other animals find a suitable home in the alpine zone, where both food and shelter are severely limited.

The only common residents are voles, marmots, and pikas. Sierra bighorn sheep may venture to these heights, but they generally prefer realms below timberline. Although many different species of birds fly through the alpine zone, the rosy finch is the only common member.

Continuing east over the Sierra Crest, below the alpine and subalpine zones, you will encounter forest zones similar to those on the west side with one major distinction. The great barrier of the Sierra Nevada insures that the precipitation falling on the **east side** of the range will be much less than what falls on the west side. Consequently, trees and plants found east of the crest have adapted to the drier conditions, which results in a more scattered forest and shorter individual trees. Trees common to the eastside montane forest include white fir, western white pine, Sierra juniper, lodgepole pine, Jeffrey pine, and incense cedar.

Below the montane forest belt, at elevations roughly between 6000 and 9000 feet, is the **pinyon-juniper woodland**, composed primarily of widely scattered, singleleaf pinyon pine, Sierra juniper, and curl-leaf mountain mahogany. These trees can withstand the dry conditions east of the crest, where only 5 to 15 inches of precipitation falls each year. Open areas are often filled with sagebrush, rabbitbrush, and bitterbrush. Many eastside trails into the High Sierra begin in this zone. Animals common to the pinyon-juniper woodland include a wide variety of amphibians, reptiles, birds, and insects. Mammals include mice, squirrels, voles, rabbits, shrews, chipmunks, coyotes, skunks, badgers, and mule deer.

When to Go: Weather and Seasons

The low-elevation foothills region of Sequoia National Park does offer some off-season hiking opportunities and one hike in this guide (Trail 1) samples this zone. **Spring** is the best time of year for the foothills, when the higher elevations are still locked in the deep freeze of winter's snowpack. During this time, foothills wildflowers are ablaze with color, the grasses are lush and green, the oaks are budding out, and temperatures are mild.

Above the foothills, snow-free hiking in the montane zone on the western side of the parks generally begins sometime in May, when the road into Kings Canyon is opened and trails in Giant Forest and Grant Grove shed winter's mantle. Once the spring thaw is underway, the snow line steadily recedes up the mountainside, opening more trails along the way. By June, most west-side paths make the frontcountry accessible, but the High Sierra typically remains buried in snow until early to mid-July, depending on the depth of the previous winter's snowpack and the late spring and early summer weather.

If you're a typical hiker using this guidebook, you'll probably visit the parks and surrounding backcountry during the **summer**. Unlike most mountain ranges in the U.S., the Sierra Nevada is summer dry, receiving only about 1.5 inches of precipitation, most of which falls from random thunderstorms. About 95 percent of the moisture that falls on the Sierra Nevada usually comes between November and March in the form of rain in the foothills and snow in the higher elevations. Summer temperatures are generally mild, although they vary considerably between the lowlands and alpine heights. By midsummer all trails in the greater Sequoia-Kings Canyon region should be snow-free, although the high passes may still hold patches of snow.

Hiking season begins in earnest during the month of July, but this period also brings a couple of concerns: Mosquitoes reach their zenith of irritation for about a two-week period and thunderstorms become a distinct possibility. Effective insect repellent, long-sleeved shirts and pants, and possibly a mosquito headnet should help to keep pesky mosquitoes at bay. If you're backpacking, be sure to include a tent with adequate mosquito netting in your pack. Thunderstorms usually occur from midafternoon until sunset but are typically short-lived and localized. However, they can be quite severe, drenching an area with wind-driven rain and shooting out bolts of lightning. When thunderheads start to develop, seek lower ground and find a spot within a large stand of forest. Avoid open areas and isolated or small groves of trees.

The first half of August generally provides the best conditions for hikers in the Sierra, as a major frontal storm (possibly with snow at the higher elevations) or an isolated thunderstorm are minimal, and the mosquito population has dwindled to the point of being only a minor irritation. Also, lakes, which typically reach maximum temperatures by late July (low to mid-70s for lower lakes and mid- to high 60s for higher lakes), are still almost as warm, providing pleasant swimming opportunities. September can often be a great time to visit the High Sierra, when the number of visitors to the parks drops dramatically after Labor Day weekend. During this period, backpackers should always check the weather forecast for possible storms. Tents are highly recommended during this time as well.

Fall can be a pleasant time for a visit to the foothills, when the heat of summer has abated and autumn provides a touch of color. Pleasant weather can oftentimes persist in the high country well into October, with chilly nights but mild daytime temperatures. However, backpackers must be prepared for the possibility of encountering the season's first storm during this time. The hiking season finally comes to a close with significant snowfall from the first major storm, usually by the end of the month, but occasionally not until sometime in November.

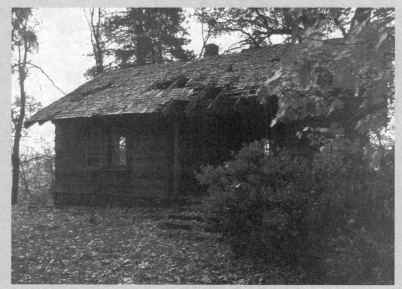

Old Colony Mill Ranger Station, *Colony Mill Road*

December ushers in the quiet **winter** season, when access along the east side of the greater Sequoia-Kings Canyon region is severely limited by snow-covered roads. However, the Park Service does a good job of maintaining access into the west side of the parks via Highway 180 and the Generals Highway, closing roads only during and immediately after substantial storms. Some lodging facilities remain open during the winter months, providing fine basecamps for cross-country skiers and snowshoers seeking to enjoy the solitude and serenity of the season without having to camp in the snow. Lodgepole Campground remains open all year, although winter campers must be prepared for snow camping. Giant Forest, Wolverton, and Grant Grove all offer marked trails for skiers and snowshoers.

Trail Selection

Several criteria were used to arrange this assortment of Sequoia and Kings Canyon's 50 best trails. Only the premier hikes were included, based upon beautiful scenery, access, trail quality, and diversity of experience. Because these trips occur in two of the nation's most magnificent national parks and two of the region's most desirable wilderness areas, most of the trails selected are highly popular, although a handful of routes should offer some level of solitude (hikers willing to step off maintained trails will find lots of lonely backcountry). Anyone fortunate enough to complete all the trips described in this guide would have a comprehensive appreciation for the natural beauty of one of the West's most scenic areas.

More than 75 percent of the trails included in this guide are classified as out-and-back trips, requiring you to retrace your steps back to the trailhead from where you started. The remaining 25 percent are loop or semiloop trips.

Features and Facilities

Top Trails books contain information about "features" for each trail, such as lakes, great views, summits, waterfalls, or wildflowers. These features are listed in the margin of each trail description. Beneath the list of features is a list of facilities, including such amenities as restrooms, nearby phones, running water, or campgrounds.

Trail Safety

Although most of the trails in this book are very obvious routes, getting lost is a remote possibility. In the granite-rich High Sierra, it can be easy to lose a trail across a lengthy stretch of bedrock when it's inadequately marked by a line of rocks or a low pile of stones, called ducks. In early season, patches of snow may obscure a route as well. Frequently noting landmarks along the way will help you to stay on route—if you find yourself uncertain about your location, simply backtrack to your last known landmark.

Elevations in the Sequoia-Kings Canyon region vary dramatically from the lowland foothills to alpine heights above 14,000 feet. Hikers who reside at or near sea level who recreate at the higher elevations in this range may experience symptoms of altitude sickness, which include headache, fatigue, loss of appetite, shortness of breath, nausea, vomiting, dizziness, drowsiness, memory loss, and loss of mental acuity. Untreated, altitude sickness may lead to the much more severe acute mountain sickness (AMS), requiring immediate medical assistance, without which victims may die.

To avoid altitude sickness, acclimatize slowly, drink plenty of fluids, and eat a diet high in carbohydrates just prior to your trip. Spending the night before your trip at a campground near the trailhead is a good way to get a jump on the acclimatization process. A rapid descent to lower elevations is usually enough to alleviate any symptoms should they develop. A severe case of AMS is unlikely in the Sierra but not impossible—AMS-caused deaths have occurred here.

Less atmosphere at higher altitudes with which to filter the sun's rays increases the risks of exposure. Always wear an appropriate sunblock on exposed skin and reapply often as necessary. Sunburns can occur even on cloudy days. A decent pair of sunglasses will protect the eyes, an especially important precaution when you're around reflective snow-covered slopes and granite bedrock.

Dehydration is another potential hazard while recreating in the back-country. Carry and drink plenty of fluids while on the trail. An electrolyte replacement drink can be quite restorative during periods of intense exertion. Check your route for water sources along the way, plan accordingly, and always filter any water acquired in the field to prevent giardia.

Although the summer weather in the High Sierra is usually fair, conditions can change radically and rapidly at any time. Pack along the appropriate gear to endure any significant climate change. Even if the weather is pleasant, temperatures can be significantly different between the trailhead and your destination. Dousing rains from thunderstorms can leave the ill prepared soaked and cold, potentially leading to hypothermia. Cold fronts have produced snow during every month of the year in the High Sierra. Lightning strikes during infrequent but not uncommon afternoon thunderstorms can be quite dangerous. If thunderclouds start to develop, do not venture above the forest cover. If you find yourself near or above treeline, beat a hasty retreat to lower elevations. Thankfully, most thunderstorms pass rather quickly in the Sierra.

The animal kingdom may provide additional safety issues. Mosquitoes can be major irritants during midsummer, when long pants, long-sleeved shirts, and mosquito netting may be good choices of apparel. These pests are most prevalent around meadows and lakeshores and in moist lodgepole pine forests. Before August, backpacking with a tent is highly advisable. Application and reapplication of an effective repellent (usually with plenty of DEET, and avoiding direct contact with your skin) should help keep the winged pests at bay when you are on the trail or in camp. Such repellent usually is effective on ticks as well, although in the High Sierra ticks are typically much less of a nuisance than mosquitoes (watch for ticks at lower elevations, particularly in spring). However, there exists the remote possibility that a tick can infect you with a number of ailments, including Lyme disease and Rocky Mountain spotted fever. When in tick country, inspect your body regularly and check your clothes for any loose bugs. If a tick bites you, use a pair of good tweezers to firmly grasp the pest, applying firm but gentle traction in order to remove the tick from your flesh, making sure not to leave the head behind. After removal, wash the affected area thoroughly with antibacterial soap and apply an antibiotic ointment. Consult a physician if flulike symptoms such as headache, rash, joint pain, or fever develop.

Black bears are the largest animals you might possibly see in the Sierra. (Grizzly bears were exterminated from the Sierra early in the 20th century.) Thanks to recent efforts by the National Park Service and U.S. Forest Service to require bear canisters in some areas and encourage their use in others, encounters between bears and humans in the backcountry has been greatly reduced (although in the last decade nine injuries have occurred and several human-food-conditioned bears were put to death). The NPS is planning to remove all backcountry food lockers and require the use of canisters everywhere in the backcountry as early as 2009. Backpackers can rent bear canisters at visitors centers and stores within the parks and at Forest Service ranger stations. Dayhikers need not worry about bear encounters, as bears usually search for food at campsites at night.

Whereas omnivorous bears see humans as bearers of food, exclusively carnivorous mountain lions, also referred to as cougars, see you as food. Therefore, avoid hiking alone and, if you have children along, keep them close by. Although the likelihood of an attack is extremely remote, if attacked you should fight back. Trying to run away is merely inviting pursuit; such behavior is exactly what prey does when threatened. Make yourself appear as large as possible, hold your ground, wave your arms, and make noise.

Nearly as remote a possibility as meeting up with a mountain lion is the likelihood of encountering a rattlesnake on the trail. The chance of being bitten is even more remote, and the odds of dying from such a bite are incredibly low. Rattlers are not aggressive and will seek an escape route unless cornered. If you happen upon one (chances are highest in the western foothills and below 6000 feet in the pinyon-juniper zone on the east side of the Sierra), quickly back away to allow the snake a safe path of escape.

The most common large animals you should expect to see are deer. While the general public seems inclined to treat these wild animals like Bambi, they are potentially dangerous (a young child was once killed in Yosemite Valley by a startled deer). All animals, big and small, within Sequoia, Kings Canyon, and the surrounding wilderness should be seen as wild. Do not attempt to touch or feed them. The survival of any animal that becomes familiar with human food is put at risk when fed by those who have learned about them from cartoons.

Marmots are generally seen as cute and furry rodents that produce a high-pitched whistle when approached. However, the marmots of Mineral King have developed a quirky and occasionally destructive tendency to munch on radiator hoses, brake lines, and fan belts. Fortunately, this odd behavior is usually confined to late spring and early summer. If you're planning an early season trip to Mineral King, check with the rangers about current conditions.

Fees, Camping, and Permits

Entrance to Sequoia and Kings Canyon national parks is subject to a fee. The most common fee is a 7-day pass costing $20 per vehicle. An annual pass is

$30 per vehicle. An America the Beautiful Pass is $80 per year and provides admission for one vehicle to all national parks, national monuments, and national recreation areas. Seniors 62 and over can purchase a lifetime pass with similar access for $10. Permanently disabled citizens or permanent residents can acquire a similar pass free with the proper documentation.

Many hikers prefer to stay in campgrounds during their visit. Information about the campgrounds nearest to a trailhead is included near the end of each trail's Finding the Trail section. During the height of the summer season, many campgrounds will be full. Only two of the Park Service campgrounds (Lodgepole and Dorst) accept reservations. The other 12 campgrounds are first-come, first-served. Approximately half of the Forest Service campgrounds surrounding the parks will accept reservations. Reservations can be made for both the park and national forest campgrounds by calling (877) 444-6777.

In addition to campgrounds, nearby resorts are also mentioned (where applicable) in each hike's Finding the Trail section. The parks offer several lodging options from rustic cabins to finely appointed hotel rooms. Reservations and information for facilities within the parks, operated by the Delaware North Company, and privately run options outside the parks can be obtained at www.nps.gov/seki/planyourvisit/lodging.htm.

Permits are not required for dayhikes. Backpackers must have a valid wilderness permit for entry into the backcountry of both the parks and wilderness areas. For overnight trips beginning in the parks, trailhead quotas are in effect from about the end of May through the end of September. Approximately 75 percent of the daily quota is available by advanced reservation between March 1 and September 15. A permit application can be downloaded from the park website (www.nps.gov/seki) and, when completed, submitted by mail (Sequoia and Kings Canyon National Parks, Wilderness Permit Reservations, 47050 Generals Highway 60, Three Rivers, CA, 93271) or fax (559-565-4239). A $15 nonrefundable fee is assessed per reservation and can be made by credit card, check, or money order. Successful applicants will receive a reservation confirmation by mail, which must then be turned into the nearest issue station to your departure trailhead for the actual wilderness permit. You must confirm or pick up the permit before 9 AM on the departure day, otherwise the permit is cancelled and becomes available for walk-ins. Free walk-in permits may be obtained after 1 PM on the day before departure, and unclaimed reserved permits become available after 9 AM on the day of departure.

For all overnight trips beginning on national forest lands, except those entering the Mt. Whitney Zone, trailhead quotas are in effect for John Muir Wilderness from May 1 through November 1 and the last Friday in June through September 15 in Golden Trout Wilderness. About 60 percent of

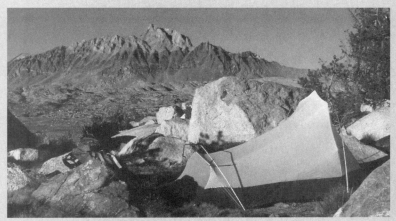

Campsite *near Mount Humphreys, Humphreys Basin (Trail 50)*

the daily quota is available by advanced reservation from six months to two days prior to the start of your trip. A permit application can be downloaded from the Inyo National Forest website (www.fs.fed.us/r5/inyo/recreation/wild/permitsres.shtml) and when completed submitted by mail (Wilderness Permit Reservation Office, 351 Pacu Lane, Suite 200, Bishop, CA 93514), fax (760-873-2484), or phone (760 873-2483). A $5 nonrefundable per person fee is assessed per reservation and can be made by credit card, check, or money order. Successful applicants will receive a reservation confirmation by mail, which must then be turned into an Inyo National Forest contact station no more than 2 days before departure to receive the actual wilderness permit. Permits must be picked up before 10 AM on the departure day, unless other arrangements are made by calling the reservation office. Free walk-in permits can be obtained starting at 11 AM the day before departure, and unclaimed advanced reservations are made available for walk-in permits after 10 AM on the day of departure.

Permits for entry into the Mt. Whitney Zone are required year-round for both dayhikes and overnight backpacks and daily quotas are in effect. Due to high demand, all permits are obtainable through a lottery process. Applications are accepted by mail beginning on February 1 and the lottery is drawn on February 15. Any remaining permits can be applied for after February 15 up to two days before the day of departure. If any leftover space remains, walk-in permits will be made available. Visit the Inyo National Forest website (www.fs.fed.us/r5/inyo) to download a lottery application and obtain more information on the lottery process.

Topographic Maps

An assortment of topographic maps at various scales cover the greater Sequoia and Kings Canyon region, as well as some specific areas within the region, such as Mt. Whitney and Mineral King. Taken along on the trail, a small-scale map covering a large area is particularly useful for identifying distant peaks, canyons, lakes, and other geographic features. The U.S. Forest Service, Tom Harrison Maps, and National Geographic Maps are good resources for maps in the Sequoia-Kings Canyon region.

I recommend that hikers and backpackers carry a more detailed map while on the trail. The 7.5-minute topographic quadrangles (1:24,000 scale) published by the U.S. Geological Survey fill this bill well. In the introductory material for each chapter under "Maps" there is a list of the pertinent USGS 7.5-minute maps needed for each trip. These maps can be ordered online at http://store.usgs.gov ($6 per map), or purchased from Forest Service or National Park Service ranger stations. Computer software that you may purchase from companies such as National Geographic (TOPO) or DeLorme allows you to customize and print topographic maps from your home computer (although the map is limited to the size of paper your printer can handle). Some outdoor retailers (REI for one) have kiosks that enable you to create and print similar maps at their stores.

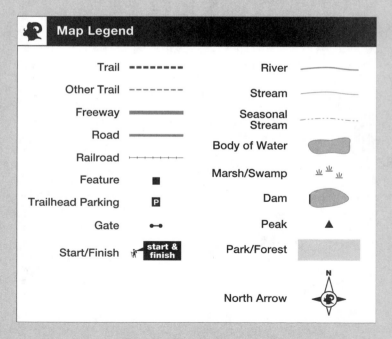

On the Trail

Every outing should begin with proper preparation, which usually takes just minutes. Even the easiest trail can turn up unexpected surprises. Hikers never think that they will get lost or suffer an injury, but accidents do happen. Simple precautions can make the difference between a good story and a dangerous situation.

Use the Top Trails ratings and descriptions to determine if a particular trail is a good match with your fitness and energy level, given current conditions and time of year. Pay particular attention to the **Best Time** description given for each trail.

Have a Plan

Choose Wisely The first step to enjoying any trail is to match the trail to your abilities. It's no use overestimating your experience or fitness—know your abilities and limitations, and use the **Top Trails Difficulty Rating** that accompanies each trail.

Leave Word The most basic of precautions is leaving word of your intentions with family or friends. Many people will hike the backcountry their entire lives without ever relying on this safety net, but establishing this simple habit is free insurance.

It's best to leave specific information—location, trail name, intended time of travel—with a responsible person. However, if this is not possible or if plans change at the last minute, you should still leave word. If there is a registration process available, make use of it. If there is a ranger station or park office, check in.

Review the Route Before embarking on any trail, be sure to read the entire description and study the map. It isn't necessary to memorize every detail, but it is worthwhile to have a clear mental picture of the trail and the general area.

If the trail and terrain are complex, augment the trail guide with a topographic map; Top Trails points out when this could be useful. Maps as well as current weather and trail condition information are often available from local ranger and park stations.

Prep and Plan

- Know your abilities and your limitations.
- Leave word about your plans.
- Know the area and the route.

Check Before Going It's a good idea to check in with the local ranger or land management agency to determine the status of the trail and the roads to the trailhead, particularly just after a storm. Roads and trails may be washed out by floods.

Carry the Essentials

Proper preparation for any type of trail use includes gathering certain essential items to carry. Trip checklists will vary tremendously by trail and conditions.

Clothing When the weather is good, light, comfortable clothing is the obvious choice. It's easy to believe that very little spare clothing is needed, but a prepared hiker has something tucked away for any emergency from a surprise shower to an unexpected overnight stay in a remote area.

Clothing includes proper footwear, essential for hiking and running trails. As a trail becomes more demanding, you will need footwear that performs. Running shoes are fine for many trails. If you will be carrying substantial weight or encountering sustained rugged terrain, step up to hiking boots.

In hot, sunny weather, proper clothing includes a hat, sunglasses, long-sleeved shirt and sunscreen. In cooler weather, particularly when it's wet, carry waterproof outer garments and quick-drying undergarments (avoid cotton). As general rule, whatever the conditions, bring layers that can be combined or removed to provide comfort and protection from the elements in a wide variety of conditions.

Also, long pants and long-sleeved shirts are a useful first line of defense against poison oak, ticks, and mosquitoes.

Water Never embark on a trail without carrying water. At all times, particularly in warm weather, adequate water is of key importance. Experts recommend at least 2 quarts of water per day, and when hiking in heat a gallon or more may be more appropriate. At the extreme, dehydration can be life threatening. More commonly, inadequate water brings fatigue and muscle aches.

For most outings, unless the day is very hot or the trail very long, you should plan to carry sufficient water for the entire trail. Unfortunately, natural water sources are usually questionable, and may be contaminated with bacteria, viruses, and other pollutants.

Water Treatment If it's necessary to make use of trailside water, you should filter or treat it. There are three methods for treating water: boiling, chemical treatment, and filtering. Boiling is best, but often impractical—it requires a heat source, a pot, and time. Chemical treatments, available in sporting goods stores, handle some problems, including the troublesome giardia parasite, but will not combat many chemical pollutants. The preferred method is filtration, which removes giardia and other contaminants and doesn't leave any unpleasant aftertaste.

If this hasn't convinced you to carry all the water you need, one final admonishment: Be prepared for surprises. Water sources described in the text or on maps can change course or dry up completely. Never run your water bottle dry in expectation of the next source; fill up when water is available and always keep a little in reserve.

Food

While not as critical as water, food is energy and its importance shouldn't be underestimated. Avoid foods that are hard to digest, such as candy bars and potato chips. Carry high-energy, fast-digesting foods: nutrition bars, dehydrated fruit, gorp, jerky. Bring a little extra food—it's good protection against an outing that turns unexpectedly long, perhaps due to weather or losing your way.

Pests and Hazards

As much as we like to think of the outdoors as our home, it can surprise us with some annoyances and pests like poison oak, ticks, mosquitoes, and rattlesnakes.

A number of the trails may support thickets of trailside poison oak. People susceptible to poison oak should wear long pants and long-sleeved shirts to avoid poison oak rash. If you suspect that poison oak has touched your skin, rinse off in a nearby stream or lake and be sure to shower as soon as you get home. Consult your doctor about treatments to help you avoid and heal from poison oak rash.

Trails may also harbor ticks lurking in the trailside vegetation. As a precaution against Lyme disease, which is spread by ticks, it is a good idea to avoid getting a tick bite by wearing a long-sleeved shirt. Tuck your pant legs

Trail Essentials

- Spare cold-weather clothing
- Plenty of water
- Adequate food (plus a little more)

into your boots. Check your appendages frequently for ticks. Wear light-colored clothing to spot ticks more easily. If you are bitten by a tick, clutch it firmly between two fingers and pull it out. Even though most ticks are not disease carriers, it is best to save the tick in a baggie or film canister. If your tick bite becomes inflamed, acquires a suspicious bull's-eye-like ring around it, or if you come down soon after the bite with flulike symptoms, consult your doctor immediately and be sure to bring the tick for identification. The long-term affects of Lyme disease can be both permanent and debilitating.

Depending on the time of the year, you may encounter mosquitoes, which can, in rare instances, carry encephalitis or the West Nile virus. But typically, you simply have to be concerned about the obnoxious itching bite of these pests. Again, a long-sleeved shirt is a good first line of defense, along with mosquito repellent.

Rattlesnakes are common on many of the Sierra foothills trails. Despite these snakes' bad rap, rattlesnake bites are rare in California, and rattlers and other snakes perform an important ecosystem function by eating rats, mice, and other small mammals that would soon strip most of the vegetation from our outdoor areas if they were not kept in check. Snakes are cold-blooded and may be found in the middle of a trail or in other open spaces sunning themselves. Just be sure to look ahead of you as you walk along a trail and be alert for the telltale rattling. Be sure to look on the other side before stepping over or sitting on logs and rocks. Rattlesnakes want nothing more than to be left alone, so avoid harassing, following, or poking at a rattler.

Attacks by mountain lions and bears on humans are very rare in California. The smaller and usually nonaggressive California black bear is more of a threat to your camping food than to anything else.

Thunderstorm-derived lightning is a concern at higher elevations. Peaks, ridgetops, and tall trees may attract lightning strikes. It's best to get to lower elevations and avoid being the highest object in your area during thunderstorms.

Less Than Essential, But Useful Items

Map and Compass (And the Know-How to Use Them) Many trails don't require much navigation, meaning a map and compass aren't always as essential as water or food—but it can be a close call. If the trail is remote or infrequently visited, a map and compass should be considered necessities. As the budgets of federal and state land management agencies have declined, so have the frequency and reliability of trail signs, as well as maintenance of the trails themselves.

A hand-held GPS receiver is also a useful trail companion, but is really no substitute for a map and compass; knowing your longitude and latitude is not much help without a map.

Cell Phone Most parts of the country, even remote destinations, have some level of cellular coverage, particularly on peaks and ridgetops. In extreme circumstances, a cell phone can be a lifesaver. But don't depend on it; coverage is unpredictable and batteries fail.

Gear Depending on the remoteness and rigor of the trail, there are many additional useful items to consider: pocketknife, flashlight, fire source (waterproof matches, lighter, or flint), and a first-aid kit. Always carry some

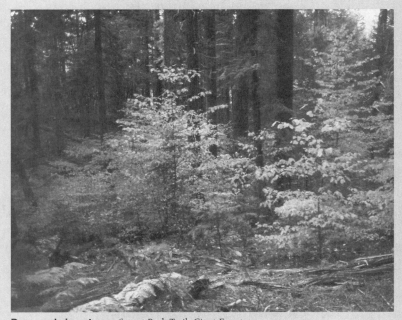

Dogwoods in autumn, *Sunset Rock Trail, Giant Forest*

Trail Etiquette

- Leave no trace—never litter.
- Stay on the trail—never cut switchbacks.
- Share the trail—use courtesy and common sense.
- Leave it there—don't disturb wildlife.

toilet paper and a light plastic trowel in case there is a need to go in the woods. Bury your waste at least 6 inches deep and more than 300 feet away from all water sources. Also, bring extra plastic bags to carry your used toilet paper out for proper disposal. A hiking staff or walking poles may enhance your experience by reducing the load on your feet and legs. Small binoculars are useful for viewing and identifying wildlife.

Every member of your party should carry the appropriate essential items described above; groups often split up or get separated along the trail. Solo hikers should be even more disciplined about preparation, and carry more gear. Traveling solo is inherently more risky. This isn't meant to discourage solo travel, simply to emphasize the need for extra preparation. Solo hikers should make a habit of carrying a little more gear than absolutely necessary.

Trail Etiquette

The overriding rule on the trail is "leave no trace." Interest in visiting natural areas continues to increase in North America, even as the quantity of unspoiled natural areas continues to shrink. These pressures make it ever more critical that we leave no trace.

Never Litter If you carried it in, it's easy enough to carry it out. Leave the trail in the same, if not better condition than you find it. Try picking up any litter you encounter and packing it out if possible.

Stay on the Trail Paths have been created, sometimes over many years, for many purposes: to protect the surrounding natural areas, to avoid dangers, and to provide the best route. Leaving the trail can cause damage that takes years to undo. Never cut switchbacks. Shortcutting rarely saves energy or time, and it takes a terrible toll on the land, trampling plant life and hastening erosion. Moreover, safety and consideration intersect on the trail. It's hard to get truly lost if you stay on the trail.

Share the Trail The best trails attract many visitors and you should be prepared to share the trail with others. Do your part to minimize impact.

Many of the trails in this book are used by hikers, mountain bikers, and equestrians. Some of the non-wilderness trails are even open to motorized use. Commonly accepted trail etiquette dictates that motor vehicles and bike riders yield to both hikers and equestrians, hikers yield to horseback riders, downhill hikers yield to uphill hikers, and everyone stays to the right. Not everyone knows these rules of the trail, so let common sense and good humor be the final guide.

Leave It There Destruction or removal of plants and animals, or historical, prehistoric, or geological items, is certainly unethical and almost always illegal.

Follow Campfire Rules Many of the higher-elevation areas are off-limits to campfires due to high use and impacts on local vegetation from wood gathering. Lower-elevation areas may have seasonal campfire prohibitions during dry periods to reduce the chance of starting a wildfire. Check with the management agency before your outing for permanent and seasonal rules.

Getting Lost If you become lost on the trail, stay on the trail. Stop and take stock of the situation. In many cases, a few minutes of calm reflection will yield a solution. Consider all the clues available; use the sun to identify directions if you don't have a compass. If you determine that you are indeed lost, remain on the main trail and stay put. You are more likely to encounter other people if you stay in one place.

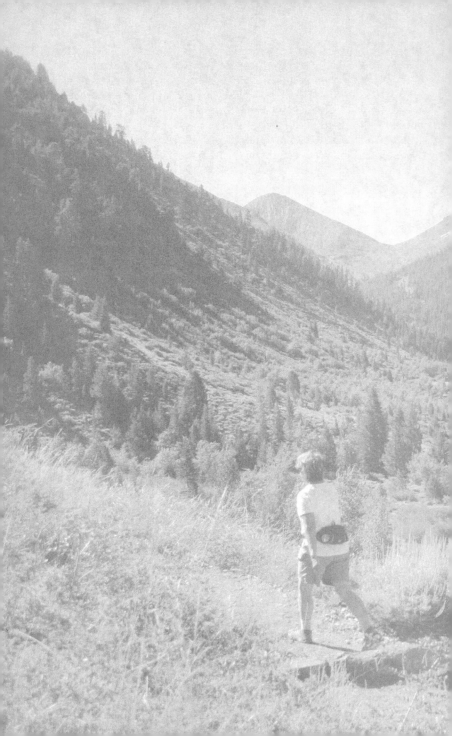

West Sequoia

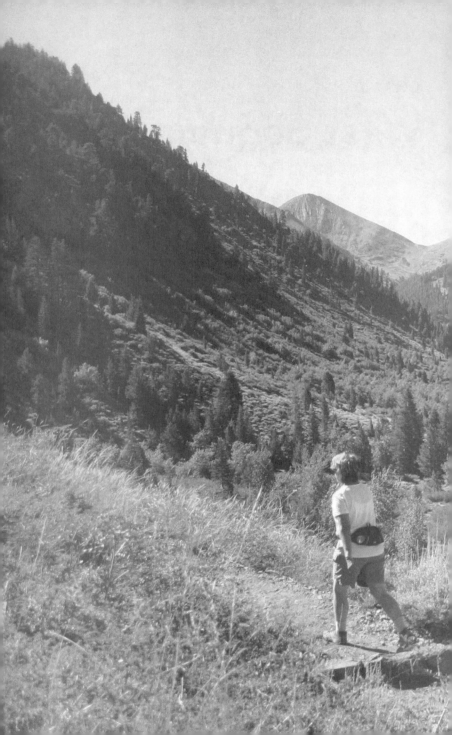

West Sequoia

The west side of the Sierra Nevada rises slowly but steadily from the broad plain of the San Joaquin Valley toward the federally protected lands of Sequoia National Park. Traveling east, the verdant and productive agricultural lands of the San Joaquin Valley gradually transition into the oak-dotted grasslands and chaparral of the foothills zone, followed by a sea of green from the dense timber of the mid-elevation forests. Fortunately, only a few roads penetrate this area of towering conifers and isolated groves of giant sequoias, and auto-bound tourists are completely blocked from access to the granite cirques, alpine meadows, and jagged peaks associated with the High Sierra. Steadily rising, roadless wilderness continues through the red fir and lodgepole pine forests into the subalpine and alpine zones before climaxing at the Sierra Crest, along the eastern border of the park.

Visitors entering Sequoia from the west experience a wide range of topography, flora, and fauna. The foothills region offers a unique opportunity to experience a slice of California's lower elevation terrain in an undeveloped setting—a definite rarity throughout most of the rest of the state. Because of the low elevations and mild weather, year-round hiking is possible along the **South Fork Kaweah and Middle Fork Kaweah rivers.**

Trail 1 follows a low-elevation trail to a pair of tributary canyons of the South Fork, a fine early season hike when the rest of the Sierra remains buried under winter's mantle. The narrow and twisting Mineral King Road provides access for Trails 2–4 into the high country around **Atwell Mill** and **Mineral King.** At one time, the alpine-looking valley of Mineral King was slated for development as a destination ski resort, which would have necessitated improving the road to highway standards. Fortunately, the area was spared this insult, and modern-day visitors can appreciate the relative serenity found on the numerous trails that radiate from Mineral King. From the Ash Mountain Entrance, the Generals Highway parallels the course of **Middle Fork Kaweah River** through the foothill zone to trailheads for Trails 5 and 6, two more low-elevation trails.

Overleaf and opposite: *Mineral King Valley*

Climbing farther up Generals Highway, Trails 7–9 sample some of the mid-elevation terrain in the Giant Forest, where visitors stand in awe of massive giant sequoias, the largest living organisms on earth. Trails 10–12 originate from trailheads at **Wolverton** and **Lodgepole,** with the first two trips leading to lakes and peaks in the heart of Sequoia's backcountry. Trail 12 is a short hike to one of the park's most dramatic waterfalls. Continuing northbound on Generals Highway, the highlight of Trail 13 is a fine view from the top of a granite dome, while a quiet grove of giant sequoias is the destination of Trail 14.

Permits

Permits are not required for dayhikes. Backpackers must obtain a wilderness permit for all overnight visits. From trips between the Thursday before Memorial Day and the last Sunday in September, permits are based on a quota system and cost $15 per party. Off-season permits are free and available by self-registration. Up to 75 percent of the quota for each trailhead can be reserved between March 1 and September 10 (applications submitted outside of these dates will not be processed). Complete and submit a downloadable application (www.nps.gov/seki) with the $15 nonrefundable fee (Visa, MasterCard, check, or money order) by mail or fax. Applications must be received before 14 days prior to the first day of a trip. Walk-in permits may be obtained after 1 PM the day before entry from the Foothills Visitors Center or the Lodgepole Wilderness Office. Unclaimed reservations become available as walk-in permits after 9 AM on the day of entry.

Maps

For West Sequoia, the USGS 7.5-minute (1:24,000 scale) topographic maps are listed below, according to which trails they're appropriate for.

Trail 1: *Dennison Peak* and *Moses Mountain*
Trail 2: *Silver City*
Trails 3–4: *Mineral King*
Trails 5–8: *Giant Forest*
Trail 9: *Giant Forest* and *Lodgepole*
Trails 10–12: *Lodgepole*
Trail 13: *Giant Forest*
Trail 14: *Muir Grove*

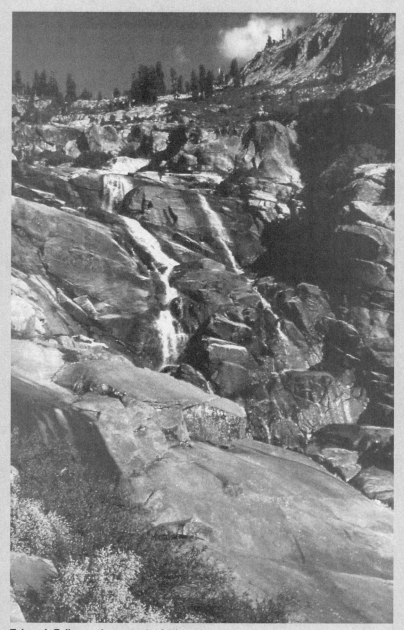

Tokopah Falls *in early summer (Trail 12)*

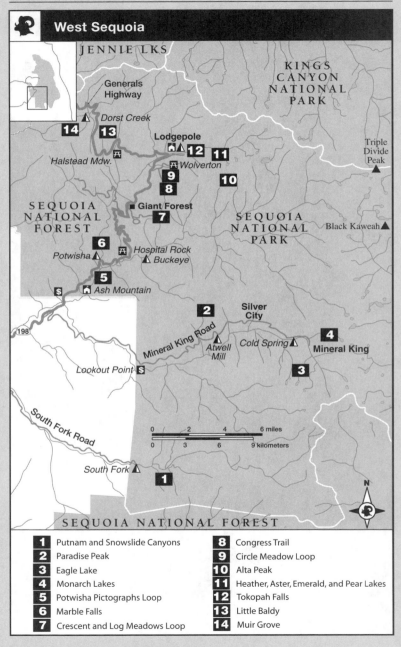

West Sequoia

JENNIE LKS

KINGS CANYON NATIONAL PARK

Generals Highway

Triple Divide Peak ▲

14 Dorst Creek

13

Lodgepole

12

11

Halstead Mdw.

Wolverton

9

10

8

SEQUOIA NATIONAL FOREST

■ Giant Forest

7

SEQUOIA NATIONAL PARK

Black Kaweah ▲

6

Hospital Rock

Potwisha ▲

▲ Buckeye

5

🏠 Ash Mountain

$

2

Silver City

4

Mineral King

198

Mineral King Road

Atwell Mill ▲

Cold Spring ▲

Lookout Point **$**

3

South Fork Road

0   2   4   6 miles
0   3   6   9 kilometers

South Fork ▲

1

N

SEQUOIA NATIONAL FOREST

1	Putnam and Snowslide Canyons	**8**	Congress Trail
2	Paradise Peak	**9**	Circle Meadow Loop
3	Eagle Lake	**10**	Alta Peak
4	Monarch Lakes	**11**	Heather, Aster, Emerald, and Pear Lakes
5	Potwisha Pictographs Loop	**12**	Tokopah Falls
6	Marble Falls	**13**	Little Baldy
7	Crescent and Log Meadows Loop	**14**	Muir Grove

TRAIL FEATURE TABLE

West Sequoia

TRAIL	Difficulty	Length	Type	USES & ACCESS	TERRAIN	FLORA & FAUNA	OTHER
1	3	6.8	Out & Back	Dayhiking, Running, Horses	Canyon, River or Stream	Wildflowers, Giant Sequoias	Great Views, Secluded
2	4	9.6	Out & Back	Dayhiking, Running, Horses	Mountain, Summit	Wildflowers, Giant Sequoias	Great Views, Secluded, Steep
3	4	6.5	Out & Back	Dayhiking, Backpacking, Running, Horses	Canyon, Lake, River or Stream	Wildflowers	Great Views, Camping, Swimming, Fishing
4	4	6.5	Out & Back	Dayhiking, Backpacking, Running, Horses	Lake, River or Stream	Wildflowers	Great Views, Camping, Swimming
5	1	0.5	Loop	Dayhiking, Child Friendly	River or Stream		Camping, Swimming, Historic Interest
6	3	6.8	Out & Back	Dayhiking	Canyon, River or Stream, Waterfall	Wildflowers	Great Views, Secluded
7	2	2.4	Loop	Dayhiking, Child Friendly		Fall Colors, Wildflowers, Giant Sequoias	Historic Interest
8	2	3.1	Loop	Dayhiking, Child Friendly		Fall Colors, Wildflowers, Giant Sequoias	
9	2	5.8	Loop	Dayhiking, Child Friendly		Fall Colors, Wildflowers, Giant Sequoias	Secluded
10	5	13.4	Out & Back	Dayhiking, Backpacking, Horses	Mountain, River or Stream	Wildflowers	Great Views, Camping, Steep
11	4	11.5	Out & Back	Dayhiking, Backpacking, Horses	Mountain, Lake	Wildflowers	Great Views, Camping, Swimming
12	2	4.1	Out & Back	Dayhiking, Horses	Canyon, Waterfall	Wildflowers	Great Views
13	3	3.5	Out & Back	Dayhiking	Mountain, Summit		Great Views
14	3	4.2	Out & Back	Dayhiking		Fall Colors, Giant Sequoias	Great Views, Secluded

Legend

USES & ACCESS
- Dayhiking
- Backpacking
- Running
- Horses
- Dogs Allowed
- Child Friendly
- Handicapped Access

TYPE
- Loop
- Out & Back

DIFFICULTY
- 1 2 3 4 5 +
less   more

TERRAIN
- Canyon
- Mountain
- Summit
- Lake
- River or Stream
- Waterfall

FLORA & FAUNA
- Fall Colors
- Wildflowers
- Giant Sequoias

FEATURES
- Great Views
- Camping
- Swimming
- Secluded
- Steep
- Historic Interest
- Fishing

West Sequoia

TRAIL 1

Dayhike, Run, Horse
6.8 miles, Out & Back
Difficulty: 3

Putnam and Snowslide Canyons..... 37

A fine early season hike to a pair of canyons above South Fork Kaweah River. Colorful wildflowers spice up early spring but the views of Homers Nose and Dennsion Mountain are excellent year-round. As with all hikes in the foothills, be on the alert for poison oak, ticks, and rattlesnakes.

TRAIL 2

Dayhike, Run, Horse
9.6 miles, Out & Back
Difficulty: 4

Paradise Peak...................... 41

A rugged climb to the top of a 9362-foot mountain is rewarded by great views. Giant sequoias in the Atwell Grove along the way provide an added bonus. Bring along plenty of water for the south-facing ascent.

TRAIL 3

Dayhike, Backpack,
Run, Horse
6.5 miles, Out & Back
Difficulty: 4

Eagle Lake 47

Perhaps the most popular hike in the Mineral King area, attractive Eagle Lake is a fine destination for those who have the stamina for it and are well acclimatized.

TRAIL 4

Dayhike, Backpack,
Run, Horse
6.5 miles, Out & Back
Difficulty: 4

Monarch Lakes..................... 53

Just about every trail out of Mineral King requires a stiff climb, and this trail to the Monarch Lakes is no exception. En route to the spectacularly scenic lakes you have splendid views of Mineral King valley bordered by dramatic-looking peaks.

Potwisha Pictographs Loop 59

This short and easy hike suitable for just about anyone leads to the banks of the Middle Fork Kaweah River, passing Native American bedrock mortars and pictographs along the way. Within the foothills zone, the trail offers the possibility of an early season hike. Later in the summer, the diminished flow in the river makes swimming an attractive proposition.

Marble Falls 63

A 3-plus-mile climb through a foothills canyon provides a year-round opportunity to stretch your legs on the way to a series of cascades known collectively as Marble Falls.

Crescent and Log Meadows Loop ... 67

Crescent Meadow is a hub of activity during the height of summer, but this short loop through a section of the Giant Forest takes you away from at least some of the crowds.

Congress Trail 73

After visiting the world's largest giant sequoia and largest living organism on the planet, the General Sherman Tree, one of the more popular trails in the Giant Forest leads to some of the more significant individual sequoias and groups of the big trees in the area. Pavement makes the trail accessible to just about anyone, and the route can be shortened by a mile round-trip by riding the free park shuttle to the General Sherman Tree bus stop.

Circle Meadow Loop 79

A longer loop trip through the Giant Forest offers an opportunity to experience the giant sequoias with a higher expectation of solitude and serenity. Visiting several named monarchs, the trail also exposes hikers to beautiful, flower-filled Circle Meadow.

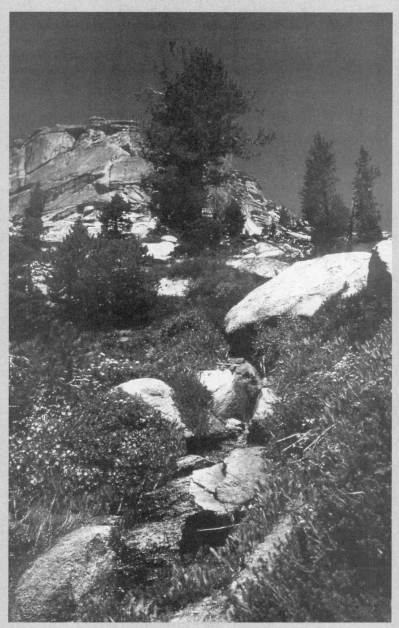

Brook below Alta Peak *(Trail 10)*

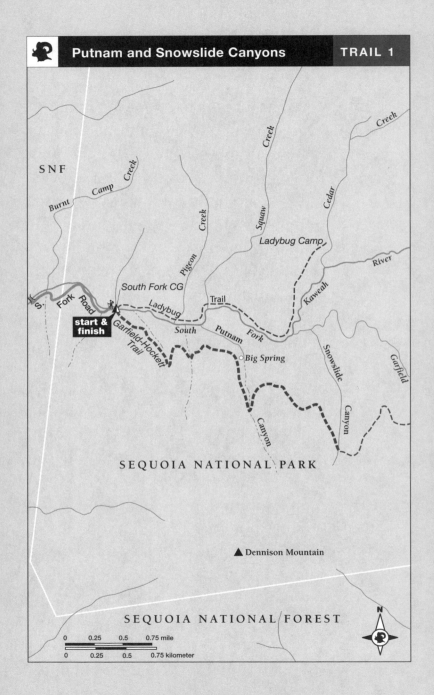

SNF

Burnt Camp Creek

South Fork Road

S. Fork Road

start & finish

Pigeon Creek

South Fork CG

Ladybug

South

Garfield-Hockett Trail

Putnam

Trail

Fork

Creek

Creek

Squaw

Ladybug Camp

River

Kaweah

Big Spring

Canyon

Snowslide Canyon

Garfield

Cedar

SEQUOIA NATIONAL PARK

▲ Dennison Mountain

SEQUOIA NATIONAL FOREST

| 0 | 0.25 | 0.5 | 0.75 mile |
| 0 | 0.25 | 0.5 | 0.75 kilometer |

N

Putnam and Snowslide Canyons

The short journey to Putnam and Snowslide canyons offers hikers early and late seas" on opportunities to enjoy the foothills zone on the western fringe of Sequoia while the higher elevations are buried in snow. Wildflowers offer splashes of color in early spring, and views of Homers Nose and Dennison Mountain are excellent throughout the hiking season. The journey to Putnam Canyon passes through oak woodland, while continuing on to Snowslide Canyon exposes hikers to a mixed coniferous forest, including a small grove of giant sequoias.

Best Time

With a location in the foothills, the first 2-plus miles of trail to Putnam Canyon can be hiked year-round. Snow may blanket the trail between Putnam Canyon and Snowslide Canyon during the winter months, but the trail should be snow-free from March to December.

Finding the Trail

Drive State Highway 198 eastbound from Visalia to the town of Three Rivers and turn right onto South Fork Road, approximately 7 miles west of the Ash Mountain Entrance. Follow South Fork Road for about 9 miles to the end of the pavement, and continue another 3 miles on narrow, dirt road to the South Fork Campground (pit toilets, no water, and no fee). Pass through the campground and leave your vehicle in the small, shady parking area.

TRAIL USE
Dayhike, Run, Horse

LENGTH
6.8 mil±±es, 3–4 hours

VERTICAL FEET
+2690/-460/±6300

DIFFICULTY
– 1 2 **3** 4 5 +

TRAIL TYPE
Out & Back

FEATURES
Canyon
Stream
Wildflowers
Giant Sequoias
Great Views
Secluded

FACILITIES
Campground

Trail Description

▶1 The signed Garfield-Hockett Trail begins at the campground access road, a short distance before the parking area. Climb moderately across an oak-dotted hillside amid lush trailside vegetation, including colorful wildflowers and a rather healthy population of poison oak. Enter a side canyon about 1 mile from the trailhead and hop across the first of many small rivulets slicing down the lower slopes of Dennison Mountain. The extra moisture in these diminutive nooks creates a dramatic change in vegetation, as ferns, thimbleberry, maples, nutmegs, alders, dogwoods, and cedars line the shady streambanks.

Continue a steady climb through oak woodland to **Putnam Canyon.**▶2 The sound of rushing water out of sight below the trail, coursing down the canyon from Big Spring, will be quite noticeable, but chances are the creek at trail level will be dry following the conclusion of snowmelt. The steep and narrow canyon is filled with boulders and low shrubs, allowing a cross-canyon view of the bulbous granite dome dubbed Homers Nose.

Beyond Putnam Canyon, the steady climb continues as a smattering of ponderosa pines, white firs, and incense cedars begin to intermix with the deciduous trees. Fortunately the arrival of the conifers coincides with the departure of the poison oak,

 Wildflowers

 Canyon

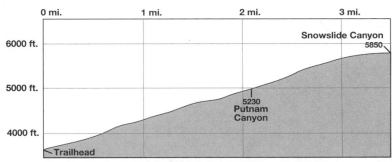

TRAIL 1 Putnam and Snowslide Canyons Elevation Profile

although the innocuous flowers and plants from the lush understory below start to disappear as well. A mile from Putnam Canyon, the oak woodland is left behind for good, as the trail bends southeast into a canyon near the western fringe of Garfield Grove. A bit farther up the trail, a dozen or so giant sequoias dwarf smaller conifers on the way to a crossing of the vigorous creek that flows down **Snowslide Canyon.▶3** Hikers will find the canyon to be a worthy early-season goal, as the winter snowpack generally covers the trail beyond here until summer.

Wildflowers offer splashes of color in early spring, and views of Homers Nose and Dennison Mountain are excellent throughout the hiking season.

👤	MILESTONES		
▶1	0.0	Start at Garfield-Hockett Trailhead	
▶2	2.1	Putnam Canyon	
▶3	3.4	Snowslide Canyon	

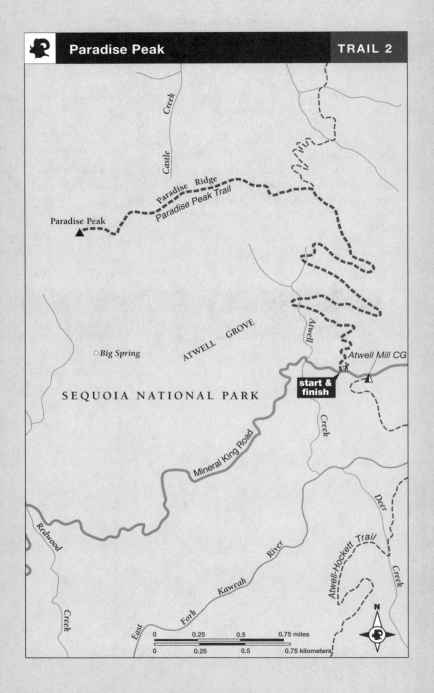

Creek

Castle

Paradise Ridge

Paradise Peak Trail

Paradise Peak ▲

Atwell

Atwell Mill CG

○ Big Spring

ATWELL GROVE

start & finish

SEQUOIA NATIONAL PARK

Creek

Mineral King Road

Deer

Redwood

Atwell-Hockett Trail

Creek

River

Kaweah

Fork

East

Creek

0	0.25	0.5	0.75 miles
0	0.25	0.5	0.75 kilometers

N

Paradise Peak

You can avoid the crowds on this nearly 10-mile hike to the top of Paradise Peak, as most recreationists willing to drive the long and winding Mineral King Road are headed farther up the road to trailheads in Mineral King valley. Additionally, the climb to the former lookout is relatively stiff, which deters even more hikers from taking this trail. However, only the first 3.75 miles are moderately steep up a south-facing slope before you gain gentler terrain along Paradise Ridge. Along the way, the Atwell Grove boasts some of the largest giant sequoias in existence. Your effort to reach the summit is well rewarded with fine views of the Great Western Divide and the surrounding foothills.

TRAIL USE
Dayhike, Run, Horse
LENGTH
9.6 miles, 4–5 hours
VERTICAL FEET
+2990/-185/±6350
DIFFICULTY
– 1 2 3 **4 5** +
TRAIL TYPE
Out & Back

FEATURES
Mountain
Summit
Wildflowers
Giant Sequoias
Great Views
Secluded
Steep

FACILITIES
Campground
Bear Box

Best Time

The Mineral King Road is usually open by Memorial Day weekend, but the trail to the top of Paradise Peak remains snowbound until mid-June and then closes with the first major storm of the season, generally in late October or early November.

Finding the Trail

Drive eastbound from Visalia on State Highway 198 to the east edge of Three Rivers and turn onto Mineral King Road. Follow the narrow and sometimes winding road to the Lookout Point Entrance Station (fee), past the entrance to Atwell Mill Campground (fee, vault toilets, running water, bear boxes, and phone), and then 0.2 mile farther to the signed trailhead parking area near the east edge of the campground, 18.2 miles from Highway 198.

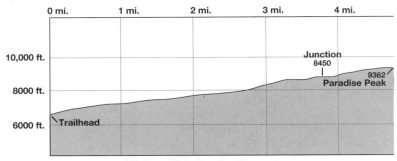

TRAIL 2 Paradise Peak Elevation Profile

Silver City Mountain Resort is a short distance up the road, offering cabins, chalets, showers, a restaurant and bakery, and a limited selection of supplies.

Trail Description

▶1 From the parking area you must head back down the Mineral King Road for a quarter mile to the signed Paradise Ridge Trailhead, where single-track trail begins a moderate climb through a mixed forest of white firs, ponderosa pines, sugar pines, incense cedars, and young sequoias shading an understory of mountain misery and manzanita. Soon a series of switchbacks lead far up the hillside past an opening in the forest, where medium-size giant sequoias make an appearance, just before a small fern-and-alder-lined seasonal rivulet. Larger sequoias will be seen farther up the trail, which are some of the 20 to 30 largest specimens in the Sierra.

Additional switchbacks lead steeply up the hillside and toward Atwell Creek—contrary to what is shown on the USGS 7.5-minute *Silver City* quadrangle, the trail approaches but does not cross the creek. If you need water after the thirst-inducing climb, you'll have to thrash your way through thick brush to this stream, which is the only reliable water source along the entire route. Away from the stream,

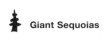
Giant Sequoias

Steep

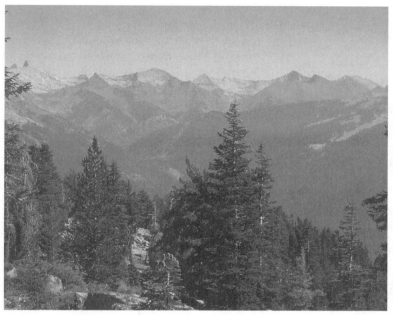

View of the Great Western Divide *from Paradise Peak*

the switchbacking ascent continues to a junction on the crest of **Paradise Ridge.▶2**

Turn west at the junction and proceed through a light forest of red firs and widely scattered patches of snowbush, chinquapin, and manzanita. The gentle grade of the trail along the ridge is a welcome respite following the steep climb up the south-facing hillside below. After passing to the north of Peak 8863, keen eyes may be able to spy the crown of the giant sequoia growing at the highest elevation in the Sierra (8800 feet) downslope to the southeast. Proceed up the ridge and then wind toward the top of the peak over rocky terrain, where distinct tread falters but the way to the summit is clear. From the summit of **Paradise Peak, ▶4** you have fine views to the east of the Great Western Divide, and to the

 Summit

Your effort to reach the summit is well rewarded with fine views of the Great Western Divide and the surrounding foothills.

north of Castle Rocks and the granite domes of Big and Little Baldy.

A trip to Paradise Peak is incomplete without experiencing the stunning view from the site of the old lookout, directly southwest of the true summit. Work your way through brush and over boulders to the base of the rock at the end of the ridge, climb some rock steps, and then scramble up a crack to the top. You may not be able to see the Great Western Divide from this vantage, thanks to a mature stand of trees, but the impressive vista to the west includes the steep cleft of Paradise Creek running into Middle Fork Kaweah River. Also visible are Moro Rock, Alta Peak, and the Generals Highway.

Paradise Peak Lookout

HISTORY

The lookout on top of **Paradise Peak** was in operation until the 1950s, when many of the fire lookouts were decommissioned in the Sierra. Nowadays, a nearby radio repeater stands as an unwelcome reminder of more contemporary human presence.

MILESTONES

▶1   0.0   Start at Paradise Peak Trailhead
▶2   3.75   Turn left (west) at junction
▶3   4.8   Summit of Paradise Peak

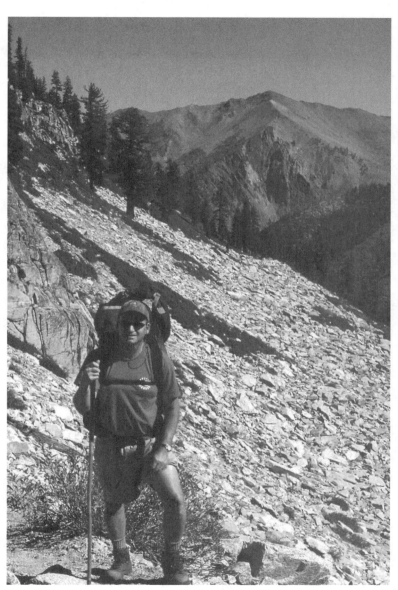

Talus Slide, *Eagle Lake Trail (Trail 3)*

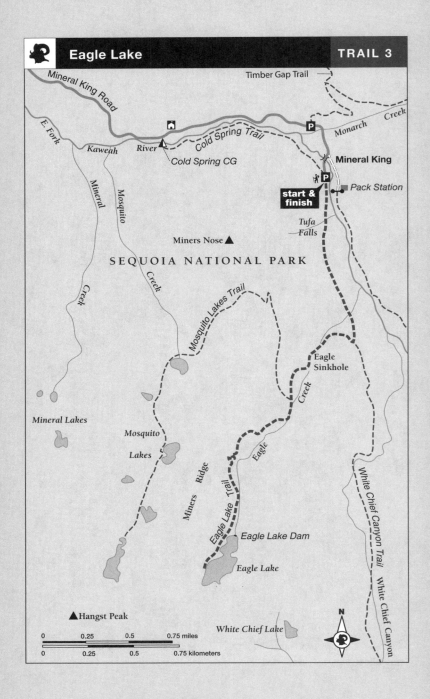

Eagle Lake

TRAIL 3

Timber Gap Trail

Mineral King Road

Monarch Creek

E. Fork

Kaweah River

Cold Spring Trail

Cold Spring CG

Mineral King

Mineral

Mosquito

Creek

Miners Nose ▲

SEQUOIA NATIONAL PARK

start & finish

Tufa Falls

Pack Station

Mosquito Lakes Trail

Eagle Sinkhole

Creek

Mineral Lakes

Mosquito

Lakes

Eagle

Miners Ridge

Eagle Lake Trail

Eagle Lake Dam

White Chief Canyon Trail

Eagle Lake

White Chief Canyon

▲Hangst Peak

| 0 | 0.25 | 0.5 | 0.75 miles |

| 0 | 0.25 | 0.5 | 0.75 kilometers |

White Chief Lake

N

Eagle Lake

Crystalline Eagle Lake, reposing majestically in a deep and scenic cirque, lures flocks of anglers, photographers, dayhikers, and backpackers to its shores seemingly every summer day. The lake's popularity is well deserved, requiring only a 3-plus-mile journey to reach, but the stiff climb demands that visitors be in reasonable physical condition. Although camping is permitted at Eagle Lake (except between the trail and the lake on the west shore) campsites are at a premium, making this trip better suited for dayhiking. Backpackers leaving cars overnight in Mineral King will need to place all food and scented items in the storage shed directly across from the ranger station, as bear boxes are not available at trailheads. Especially in early season, marmots in the area have been known to nibble on radiator hoses, fan belts, brake lines, and even radiators—check with park rangers for current conditions.

Best Time

The Mineral King Road is usually open by Memorial Day weekend, but the trail to Eagle Lake is generally snowbound until early July following winters of average snowfall. Trail use is highest from mid-July through August. The weather in September can be quite enjoyable, but Eagle Lake becomes less attractive as the water level drops by late summer.

Finding the Trail

Drive eastbound from Visalia on State Highway 198 to the east edge of Three Rivers and turn onto

TRAIL USE
Dayhike, Backpack, Run, Horse

LENGTH
6.5 miles, 3–4 hours

VERTICAL FEET
+2285/-55/±4680

DIFFICULTY
– 1 2 3 **4** 5 +

TRAIL TYPE
Out & Back

FEATURES
Mountain
Lake
Stream
Wildflowers
Great Views
Camping
Swimming
Fishing

FACILITIES
Campground
Ranger Station

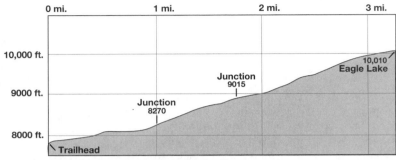

TRAIL 3 Eagle Lake Elevation Profile

Mineral King Road. Follow the narrow and sometimes winding road to the Lookout Point Entrance Station (fee) and proceed through the tiny resort community of Silver City. Silver City Mountain Resort offers cabins, chalets, showers, a restaurant and bakery, and a limited selection of supplies.

Continue past the entrance to Cold Spring Campground (fee, vault toilets, running water, bear boxes, and phone) and the Mineral King Ranger Station to the Mosquito-Eagle Trailhead at the end of the road, 23.5 miles from Highway 198. Plan on a minimum of 1¼ hours for the drive along the Mineral King Road.

The stunning scenery of Eagle Lake's steep-walled cirque is complemented by the soaring summit of Eagle Crest.

Logistics

Backpackers must obtain a wilderness permit for all overnight visits. See page 28 for more details about how to obtain one.

Trail Description

►1 South of the parking area a dirt road begins near the trailhead signboard and the restored Honeymoon Cabin. Follow this road on a mild climb up the **East Fork Kaweah River canyon** through open vegetation, sprinkled with red firs, mountain maples, and an occasional juniper. After a quarter mile, cross a removable wood bridge over Spring Creek and soon pass a lateral descending to the west bank of the river. Across the valley, cascading Crystal Creek can be seen plummeting down the far canyon wall. A mile from the trailhead, you hop across willow-lined **Stream** Eagle Creek and shortly arrive at a signed **junction** with the White Chief Canyon Trail.▶2

Follow the trail around a hillside to a set of steep switchbacks climbing through pockets of meadow alternating with stands of red firs and lodgepole pines. The grade eases on the approach to Eagle Sinkhole, where a stretch of Eagle Creek mysteriously disappears on a temporarily subterranean course. The ascent resumes past this anomaly, soon leading to a **junction** with the trail to Mosquito Lakes.▶3

From the junction, the trail climbs mildly alongside Eagle Creek to the far end of a meadow, where a steeper, switchbacking ascent leads up a forested hillside and then to the base of an expansive, talus-littered slope. A long, ascending traverse across the talus heads toward the lip of Eagle Lake's basin, with fine views of Mineral Peak, Sawtooth Peak, and the silvery thread of cascading Crystal Creek along the way. The grade eases past the talus, as you pass through pockets of grasses and shrubs, and

HISTORY

Eagle Lake Dam

The Mt. Whitney Power and Electric Company built the dam at **Eagle Lake** in the early 1900s, to regulate water flow for power production at a downstream generating plant in Hammond. Similar dams were constructed nearby at Crystal, Franklin, and Monarch lakes. Today, the water in Eagle Lake is regulated by Southern California Edison Company, resulting in a dramatic drop in lake level by late season, which has a tendency to diminish the attractiveness of the lake toward the end of summer.

Lake

Great Views

Camping

scattered boulders and rock slabs beneath a light forest of lodgepole pines. A short section of steeper climbing leads to the concrete dam at the north end of **Eagle Lake.▶4**

The stunning scenery of Eagle Lake's steep-walled cirque is complemented by the soaring summit of Eagle Crest immediately to the south. Opposite, a row of multicolored peaks rim the deep cleft of Mineral King. Just beyond the dam, a lateral heads uphill a short distance to a screened pit toilet, placed here by the Park Service in hopes of minimizing the pollution generated at this popular destination. Camping is not allowed between the trail and the lake, with the best sites for overnight accommodations about midway down the west shore. Anglers may enjoy fishing for small to medium brook trout.

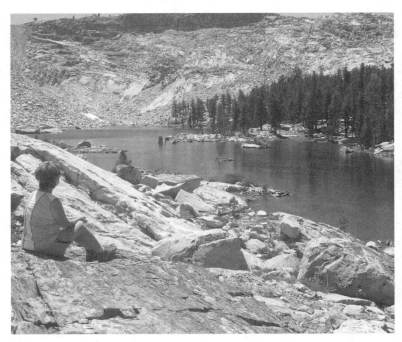

Eagle Lake

OPTIONS

Mosquito Lakes Cross-Country Route

Off-trail enthusiasts can ascend Miners Ridge to the west and then drop down to the Mosquito Lakes basin. The route is short but quite steep, with a particularly rocky descent on the Mosquito Lakes side. The least difficult crossing is directly upslope from the Eagle Lake Dam. Once at Mosquito Lake #4 (around 9910 feet in elevation), you could work your way cross-country down-canyon to pick up an unmaintained path to Mosquito Lake #1, where distinct and maintained tread leads 1.5 miles back to the junction with the Eagle Lake Trail. From there, retrace your steps 1.75 miles to the Mosquito-Eagle Trailhead. Plan on an hour or two extra for this diversion.

MILESTONES

- ►1   0.0   Start at Mosquito-Eagle Trailhead
- ►2   1.0   Turn right (south) at White Chief Canyon junction
- ►3   1.75   Proceed straight ahead (south-southwest) at Mosquito Lakes junction
- ►4   3.25   Eagle Lake

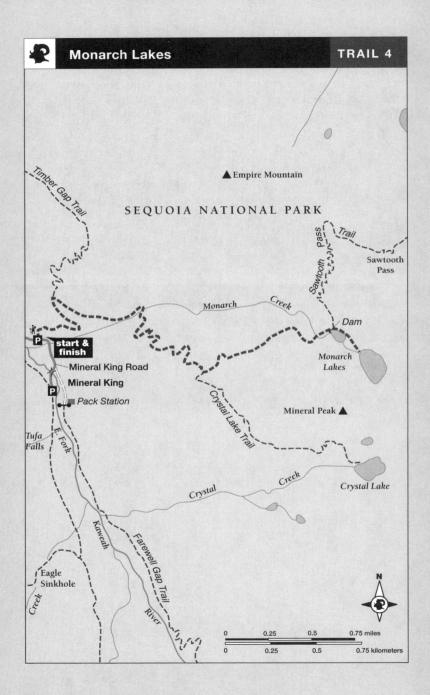

▲ Empire Mountain

SEQUOIA NATIONAL PARK

Timber Gap Trail

Sawtooth Pass Trail

Sawtooth Pass

Monarch Creek

Dam

Monarch Lakes

P

start & finish

Mineral King Road

Mineral King

P

Pack Station

Crystal Lake Trail

Mineral Peak ▲

Tufa Falls

E. Fork

Crystal Creek

Crystal Lake

Crystal

Kaweah

Farewell Gap Trail

Eagle Sinkhole

Creek

River

N

| 0 | 0.25 | 0.5 | 0.75 miles |
| 0 | 0.25 | 0.5 | 0.75 kilometers |

Monarch Lakes

The reward for this hike's stiff climb is a pair of picturesque subalpine lakes cradled in a dramatic cirque basin beneath multicolored peaks of metamorphic rock. Not only is the destination stunningly beautiful, but the vistas of the Mineral King area during the ascent are equally impressive. Despite the climb—2500 feet in 3-plus miles—the trip up the Sawtooth Pass Trail is popular with backpackers and dayhikers alike.

Since the overused campsites become cramped during peak season, you may want to view this trip as a dayhike only. If you insist on camping, don't expect a lot of peace and quiet. Backpackers leaving cars overnight in Mineral King need to place all food and scented items in the storage shed directly across from the ranger station, as bear boxes are not available at trailheads. Especially in early season, marmots in the area have been known to nibble on radiator hoses, fan belts, brake lines, and even radiators—check with park rangers for current conditions.

Best Time

The Mineral King Road is usually open by Memorial Day weekend, but the trail to Monarch Lakes is usually snowbound until early July following winters of average snowfall. Trail use is highest from mid-July through August. The weather in September can be quite enjoyable.

TRAIL USE
Dayhike, Backpack, Run, Horse

LENGTH
6.5 miles, 3–4 hours

VERTICAL FEET
+2740/-400/±6280

DIFFICULTY
– 1 2 3 **4** 5 +

TRAIL TYPE
Out & Back

FEATURES
Lake
Stream
Wildflowers
Great Views
Camping
Swimming

FACILITIES
Campground
Ranger Station
Bear Box

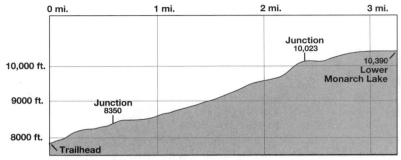

TRAIL 4 Monarch Lakes Elevation Profile

Finding the Trailhead

Drive eastbound from Visalia on State Highway 198 to the east edge of Three Rivers and turn onto Mineral King Road. Follow the narrow and sometimes winding road to the Lookout Point Entrance Station (fee) and proceed through the tiny resort community of Silver City. Silver City Mountain Resort offers cabins, chalets, showers, a restaurant and bakery, and a limited selection of supplies.

Continue past the entrance to Cold Spring Campground (fee, vault toilets, running water, bear boxes, and phone) and the Mineral King Ranger Station to the Sawtooth-Monarch Trailhead, 0.8 mile from the ranger station and 23 miles from Highway 198.

Logistics

Backpackers must obtain a wilderness permit for all overnight visits. See page 28 for more details about how to obtain one.

Trail Description

 Steep

▶1 A steep climb leads away from the trailhead up a hillside covered with sagebrush, manzanita, and gooseberry for 0.6 mile to a junction with the **Timber Gap Trail** ▶2 heading north toward Timber Gap.

Turn right at the junction and continue southeast on the Sawtooth Pass Trail, as more reasonably graded trail follows long-legged switchbacks up the hillside to Groundhog Meadow, slightly misnamed for the ubiquitous yellow-bellied marmot, a relative of the eastern woodchuck, that inhabits the meadows and rocky slopes of the subalpine Sierra. Near the meadow, you hop across sparkling Crystal Creek and begin a series of lengthy switchbacks leading in and out of shady red fir forest on the way to a junction with the seldom-used **Crystal Lake Trail.** ▶3

Veer left (northeast) at the junction and continue climbing up the Sawtooth Pass Trail. After a pair of switchbacks, cross a minor ridge at the edge of expansive and rock-strewn Chihuahua Bowl and begin a mildly ascending traverse across a barren, austere rock slope well above the level of Monarch Creek coursing through the deep cleft below. Eventually, the trail curves toward more hospitable looking terrain again, meeting the meadow-lined creek just below the outlet of **Lower Monarch Lake** and ascending shortly to the west side of the lake. ▶4 Sandwiched between multihued Sawtooth and Mineral peaks on the Great Western Divide, the two Monarch Lakes nestle picturesquely in a scenic cirque basin. Scratched out of the rocky

Sandwiched between multihued Sawtooth and Mineral peaks on the Great Western Divide, the two Monarch Lakes nestle picturesquely in a scenic cirque basin.

 Lake

Upper Monarch Lake Dam

NOTE

Upper Monarch Lake was dammed in the early 1900s by the Mt. Whitney Power and Electric Company to regulate water flow for power production at a generating plant downstream in Hammond. Similar dams were constructed nearby at Crystal, Franklin, and Eagle lakes. Today, the water in these lakes is regulated by Southern California Edison Company.

Camping

slopes to the west of the lakes are exposed, over-used campsites with a couple of bear boxes and a partially screened toilet nearby.

To reach the upper lake, find a use trail near the inlet amid a patch of willows and follow it up a steep hillside to larger **Upper Monarch Lake**. As most hikers go no farther than the lower lake, the upper lake offers a reasonable expectation of solitude away from the well-traveled Sawtooth Pass Trail.

OPTIONS

Cross-Country Route to Crystal Lakes

A steep but relatively straightforward off-trail route connects the Monarch Lakes with Crystal Lake. From Upper Monarch Lake, head south and ascend a steep chute to a saddle at around 11,170 feet, descend toward the tarn below, and then proceed on a short use trail down to Crystal Lake. To return to the trailhead, follow maintained trail from Crystal Lake west and then northwest on a 1.4-mile moderately steep descent over the west ridge of Mineral Peak and across Chihuahua Bowl to the junction with the Sawtooth Pass Trail. From there, retrace your steps 2.4 miles to the trailhead. Plan on an extra hour or two for this diversion.

MILESTONES

▶1	0.0	Start at Sawtooth-Monarch Trailhead
▶2	0.6	Turn right (southeast) at Timber Gap junction
▶3	2.4	Veer left (northeast) at Crystal Lake junction
▶4	3.25	Lower Monarch Lake

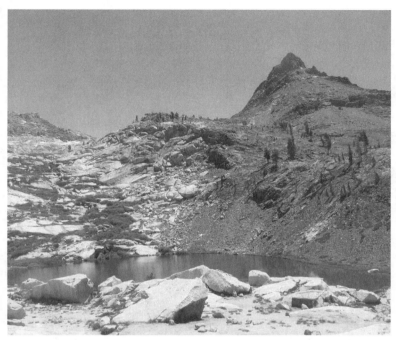

Lower Monarch Lake

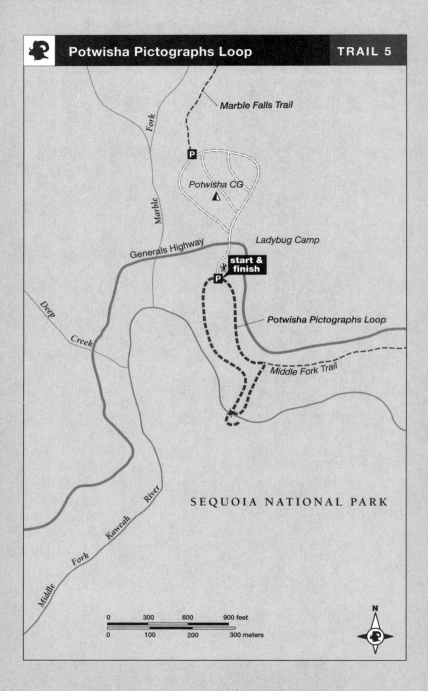

Potwisha Pictographs Loop — TRAIL 5

Marble Falls Trail

P

Potwisha CG

Generals Highway

Ladybug Camp

start & finish

P

Potwisha Pictographs Loop

Middle Fork Trail

Fork

Marble

Deep

Creek

Middle

Fork

Kaweah

River

SEQUOIA NATIONAL PARK

0   300   600   900 feet
0   100   200   300 meters

N

Potwisha Pictographs Loop

Although the Potwisha Pictographs Loop is not much of a hike by most standards, visitors of all ages will enjoy this very short trip to the banks of Middle Fork Kaweah River and back. The easy half-mile jaunt leads past a fine display of Native American bedrock mortars and pictographs, where women of the Monache tribe ground nuts and seeds and left behind pictorial representations of their culture. During the warmer months, sandy beaches and granite slabs along the picturesque river offer swimmers and sunbathers a fine haven, where the waters of the Middle Fork glide over slabs, tumble through cataracts, and swirl through delightful pools. A wood suspension bridge over the river is of special interest to the young and young at heart, although children should be closely supervised at all times, as the river can be quite treacherous when swollen with snowmelt from the mountains above.

TRAIL USE
Dayhike, Child Friendly

LENGTH
0.5 mile, ½ hour

VERTICAL FEET
+200/-200/±400

DIFFICULTY
– **1** 2 3 4 5 +

TRAIL TYPE
Loop

FEATURES
Stream
Camping
Swimming
Historic Interest

FACILITIES
Campground

Best Time

Within the foothills zone, the Potwisha Loop can be hiked year-round, although hikers will find the most pleasant conditions in spring, when temperatures are mild, the grasses are green, and the wildflowers are in bloom. Afternoon temperatures are quite hot during the summer months, when the flow of the Kaweah River is usually safe enough for a refreshing swim.

Bedrock Mortars

The Monache used bedrock mortars to grind acorns from the native oak trees into meal, a staple of their diet. Since only females were involved in this activity, anthropologists assume female members of the tribe drew the nearby pictographs, the meanings of which remain a mystery.

Finding the Trail

The easy half-mile jaunt leads past a fine display of Native American bedrock mortars and pictographs.

From Visalia, follow Highway 198 to Three Rivers and proceed east into Sequoia National Park, where the road becomes Generals Highway. Follow Generals Highway for 3.8 miles past the Ash Mountain Entrance to Potwisha Campground (fee, flush toilets, running water, bear boxes, and phone). Rather than turning left into the campground, turn right toward the campground dump station. Instead of continuing down the dump station loop toward the Middle Fork trailhead, follow the gravel surface to the end of a broad clearing above the river and park near some trash bins, where a path heads down toward the river.

Trail Description

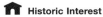

Historic Interest

▶1 Descend along a path toward **Middle Fork Kaweah River,** soon arriving near a series of granite slabs, site of numerous Native American bedrock mortars. An overhanging rock to the south has several pictographs on the underside surface.

Leaving the mortars and pictographs behind, continue across a slope dotted with granite boulders toward the river and a **wood suspension bridge.**▶2 Cross the bridge to granite slabs on the far bank, which provide excellent views of the pools and cataracts of the Middle Fork and offer fine spots on a warm summer day for sunbathing after a refreshing

dip in the water. Swimmers should exercise caution 🏊• **Swimming**
here, as the turbulent waters of the Middle Fork can
be quite hazardous when the river is running swift
and high. The path quickly dead-ends above the
bridge near an old flume.

Once you've enjoyed this pleasant site to the
fullest, retrace your steps across the bridge and
veer to the right on a path heading toward a large-
diameter steel pipe. Faint tread follows the pipe on
a short, steep climb up the hillside to an informal
junction with the Middle Fork Trail. Turn left at the
junction and follow the trail high above the level of
the river through typical oak woodland back to the
dump station parking area. From there, walk across
the gravel parking area to your car. ▶3

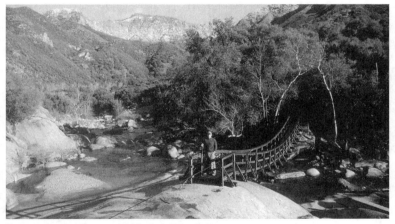

Suspension bridge *over Middle Fork Kaweah River*

🚶	MILESTONES		
▶1	0.0	Start at trailhead
▶2	0.25	Bridge over Middle Fork Kaweah River
▶3	0.5	Return to trailhead

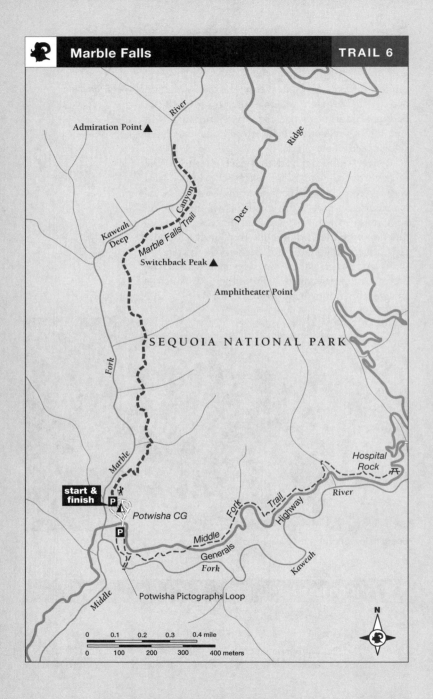

River

Ridge

Admiration Point ▲

Canyon

Deer

Kaweah
Deep

Marble Falls Trail

Switchback Peak ▲

Amphitheater Point

SEQUOIA NATIONAL PARK

Fork

Marble

Hospital
Rock

start &
finish   P

P   Trail   River

Potwisha CG   Highway

Fork

Middle

Generals   Kaweah

Fork

Middle

Potwisha Pictographs Loop

N

0	0.1	0.2	0.3	0.4 mile
0	100	200	300	400 meters

Marble Falls

A year-round hiking opportunity, Marble Falls is especially delightful in spring, when the Marble Fork Kaweah River tumbles down marble-filled Deep Canyon in full regalia and the High Sierra is still cloaked in winter's mantle. The waterfalls are not the only delights this trail offers in springtime, as patches of verdant meadow grass and an assortment of vibrant wildflowers provide an added bonus. Hiking in the foothills zone does pose a trio of concerns uncommon in the high country, namely ticks, poison oak, and rattlesnakes, although they should be more than manageable with the proper precautions.

Best Time

For this all-year hike in the foothills zone of west Sequoia, the conditions are best from March to May when the falls are at peak glory.

Finding the Trail

From Visalia, follow Highway 198 to Three Rivers and proceed east into Sequoia National Park, where the road becomes Generals Highway. Follow Generals Highway for 3.8 miles past the Ash Mountain Entrance to Potwisha Campground (fee, flush toilets, running water, bear boxes, and phone) and turn left into the campground. Follow the loop through the campground to the dirt access road at the northwest end; turn up this short road and park in the small parking area.

TRAIL USE
Dayhike

LENGTH
6.8 miles, 3–4 hours

VERTICAL FEET
+1750/-300/±4100

DIFFICULTY
– 1 2 **3** 4 5 +

TRAIL TYPE
Out & Back

FEATURES
Canyon
Stream
Waterfall
Wildflowers
Great Views
Secluded

FACILITIES
Campground

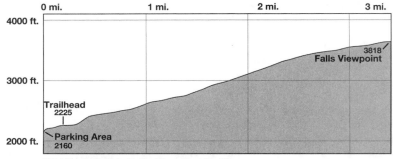

TRAIL 6 Marble Falls Elevation Profile

Trail Description

▶1 From the parking area, walk up the continuation of the dirt road to a wood plank bridge spanning a concrete-lined flume, cross the bridge, and then continue up the road on the far side to a stream flow gauge and a fenced control gate. The signed **Marble Falls Trail** begins opposite the gate. ▶2

Leave the road behind and start climbing moderately via switchbacks across a hillside dotted with typical foothill woodland trees and brilliant wildflowers in spring. Be on the alert for poison oak, which is prevalent along the initial stretch of trail. Beyond the switchbacks the trees are left behind and replaced by chaparral, as the trail climbs high above the Marble Fork around ridges and through seams on the east side of **Deep Canyon.** The chaparral-covered slopes allow views down the turbulent Middle Fork, which are briefly interrupted by short forays into small woodland groves lining the crossings of numerous rivulets and seasonal swales on the way up the canyon. The **Marble Fork** provides dramatic scenery in spring, when the swollen watercourse cascades over rock steps and swirls through churning pools, producing a raucous thunder reverberating between the walls of the deep canyon. Continue the climb up the east side of the canyon to the last stream crossing, which drains the south-

The Marble Fork provides dramatic scenery in spring, when the swollen watercourse cascades over rock steps and swirls through churning pools.

 Stream

west slope of Switchback Peak. Amid woodland, you wrap back around into the main canyon and climb across a hillside to meet the river, where the trail abruptly ends amid a **jumble of boulders and steep slabs** that inhibit further progress. ▶3

Although the name "Marble Falls" specifically applies to the uppermost fall in Deep Canyon, which is hidden from sight by the steep canyon walls, a collective series of picturesque falls visible from the end of the trail will delight visitors. Across the cleft, Admiration Point stands guard over the thunderous clamor the water creates, spilling over glistening marble precipices into wildly churning pools. The most accessible vantage point is just down from the end of the trail, where short paths lead to impressive views from thin grassy benches above the lower falls. By scrambling over boulders, angled slabs, and steep sections of canyon wall, you could make limited progress up-canyon to more views, but the terrain becomes quite treacherous—this off-trail route should be attempted only by adventurers skilled in such travel. The terrain becomes even more difficult farther up-canyon.

 Waterfall

 Great Views

🚶	**MILESTONES**	
▶1	0.0	Start at parking area
▶2	0.2	Trailhead
▶3	3.4	Viewpoint

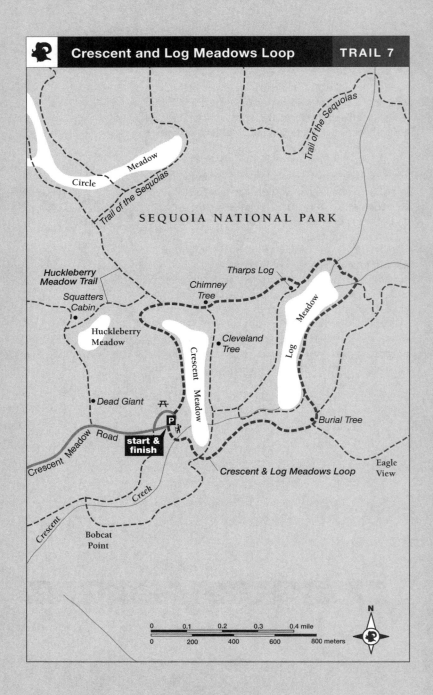

SEQUOIA NATIONAL PARK

Trail of the Sequoias

Circle   Meadow

Huckleberry
Meadow Trail

Squatters
Cabin

Huckleberry
Meadow

Tharps Log

Chimney
Tree

Cleveland
Tree

Log
Meadow

Crescent
Meadow

Dead Giant

P

start &
finish

Crescent Meadow Road

Crescent

Creek

Bobcat
Point

Burial Tree

Crescent & Log Meadows Loop

Eagle
View

N

0	0.1	0.2	0.3	0.4 mile
0	200	400	600	800 meters

Crescent and Log Meadows Loop

The Crescent Meadow area is one of the busiest spots in Sequoia National Park. Despite the potential crowds, this short journey to two flower-filled meadows and numerous majestic giant sequoias is a must-do trip for any visitor to the Giant Forest. A stop at Tharps Log completes the quintessential experience.

Best Time

Trails in Giant Forest are generally snow-free by the first part of June and remain so usually until sometime in November. Summer is by far the busiest time, when parking spaces are at a premium—consider riding the free shuttle bus during peak season. The best time to view the verdant sedges and grasses of Crescent and Log meadows is midsummer, when they're complemented by a palette of color from a copious variety of wildflowers. Autumn can be a fine time for a visit as well, especially when crowds are small and the dogwoods are ablaze with fall color.

Finding the Trail

From Visalia, follow Highway 198 to Three Rivers and proceed east into Sequoia National Park, where the road becomes Generals Highway. Drive Generals Highway to the Giant Forest Museum. Either park your vehicle in the large parking lot and ride the free shuttle bus, or drive along the narrow Crescent Meadow Road 1.2 miles to the Moro Rock junction. Motorists should continue on the Crescent

TRAIL USE
Dayhike, Child Friendly

LENGTH
2.4 miles, 1½ hours

VERTICAL FEET
+450/-450/±900

DIFFICULTY
– 1 **2** 3 4 5 +

TRAIL TYPE
Loop

FEATURES
Fall Colors
Wildflowers
Giant Sequoias
Historic Interest

FACILITIES
Restrooms
Water
Picnic Area
Shuttle Bus Stop

Meadow Road another 1.3 miles to the end of the road at the Crescent Meadow parking lot. Lodgepole is the nearest campground, about 9 miles away via Generals Highway from the Giant Forest Museum (fee, flush toilets, running water, bear boxes, and phone). Wuksachi Village, a short distance north of Lodgepole, offers upscale lodging and dining.

Trail Description

▶1 Begin your journey by following the famed High Sierra Trail, a 60-plus-mile path connecting the big trees (giant sequoias) with the big mountain (Mt. Whitney). This fabled path begins as a paved trail that crosses a pair of short wood bridges over Crescent Creek and then passes junctions with the **Crescent Creek** and **Bobcat Point trails.** ▶2 Beyond the second junction, the trail turns to dirt and makes a mild ascent across the north side of a low hill. Pass a few scattered sequoias on the way to a fork in the trail in a forested saddle near the Burial Tree. ▶3

Descend northwest from the junction, soon dropping to another junction near the southeast edge of **Log Meadow,** ▶4 a grass-and-flower-filled glade ringed by giant sequoias and lesser conifers.

 Wildflowers

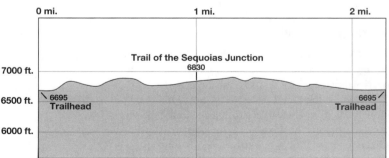

TRAIL 7 Crescent and Log Meadows Loop Elevation Profile

Tharps Log

Gaining an accurate sense of the magnitude of a mature giant sequoia is often difficult when the tree is still standing. When one of the old giants topples and stretches across the forest floor, a better perspective is gained on the true immensity of these big trees. **Tharps Log** is just such an example, large enough for the fire-hollowed interior to have been used for a summer cabin in the late 1800s. Modern-day visitors can view the restored cabin, complete with rock fireplace, bed, table, and rough-hewn benches and chairs. Interpretive signs provide some history associated with the tree, as well as a warning for visitors to respect the historical nature of the structure by remaining outside.

Hale D. Tharp, a Michigan native, settled near Three Rivers in 1856, where he quickly befriended the native Yokuts, who told their new friend of the giant trees. Two years later, Tharp was taken by the Yokuts to the Giant Forest and was later credited as being the first white man to see the big trees. Tharp later homesteaded **Log Meadow,** where he ran cattle. He used the log as a summer cabin from 1861 to 1890. Tharps Log remains the oldest human-made edifice in the park.

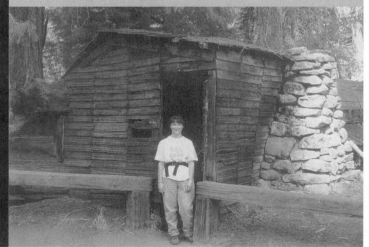

Hiker *at Tharps Log*

Crystal Cave

Many consider a trip to Sequoia National Park incomplete without a visit to magnificent **Crystal Cave**, where sweater- or jacket-clad visitors take guided tours from early May to late September to such notable features as stalactites and curtains, large cathedral-like rooms, and areas of elaborately polished marble. After purchasing advance tickets at either the Foothills or Lodgepole visitor centers (tickets are not available at the cave), a 6-plus-mile, scenic drive from Generals Highway is followed by a half-mile stroll down to the cave entrance. From there, paid ticket holders are guided on the Regular Tour (45 minutes, 50-person limit, $11 in 2009), or the Discovery Tour (1½ hours, 16-person limit, $18.95 in 2009). Spelunkers have the added opportunity to make arrangements for a 6-hour tour off the beaten path on the Wild Cave Tour ($129 in 2009, 16 years or older). For tour times or more information, contact the Sequoia Natural History Association by phone at (559) 565-3759 or by email at snha@sequoiahistory.org.

Fall Colors

Head north from the junction and walk along the east side of Log Meadow through an understory of azaleas and ferns beneath mixed forest cover. Near the north end of this lovely dell, you reach a signed T-junction with the **Trail of the Sequoias. ►5**

Proceed ahead from the junction, step over a sliver of a stream to a forested flat, and then come almost immediately to a second stream crossing on a wood plank bridge. Nearby, a number of stately sequoias line the drainage. Heading west around the northern fringe of Log Meadow, you soon reach

Historic Interest

Tharps Log, lying in a pastoral clearing, and a junction with the designated **Crescent and Log Meadows Loop. ►6**

Turn north and follow signed directions toward the Chimney Tree on the shared course of the Trail of the Sequoias and Crescent and Log Meadows Loop, climbing away from Log Meadow and soon ascending a set of stairs hewn out of a fallen sequoia.

At the top of the climb, the trail crosses a low divide separating Log and Crescent meadows. Drop off the divide on a mild descent to a pair of junctions. At the first, a very short lateral leads to the base of the Chimney Tree, where hikers can stand inside the fire-hollowed snag of a dead sequoia. This giant apparently met its doom at the hands of a fire set by a careless camper in 1919. About 25 feet farther is a second junction, ▶7 where a quick detour on the left-hand trail leads shortly to the **Cleveland Tree,** one of the larger sequoias in the Giant Forest.

 Giant Sequoias

Veer right at the second junction and skirt around the north side of **Crescent Meadow** on a short stroll through the forest to a Y-junction, where the Trail of the Sequoias heads northwest. ▶8 Turn left (southwest) and follow the west side of picturesque Crescent Meadow a half mile back to the parking lot. ▶9

🚶 MILESTONES

▶1	0.0	Start at High Sierra Trailhead
▶2	0.15	Straight at Crescent Creek and Bobcat Point junctions
▶3	0.5	Turn left (northwest) at junction near Burial Tree
▶4	0.6	Veer right (north) at junction near Log Meadow
▶5	1.1	Straight at Trail of the Sequoias
▶6	1.2	Turn right (north) at Tharps Log junction
▶7	1.5	Veer right (northwest) at second junction near Chimney Tree
▶8	1.7	Turn left (southwest) at junction of Trail of the Sequoias
▶9	2.4	Return to trailhead

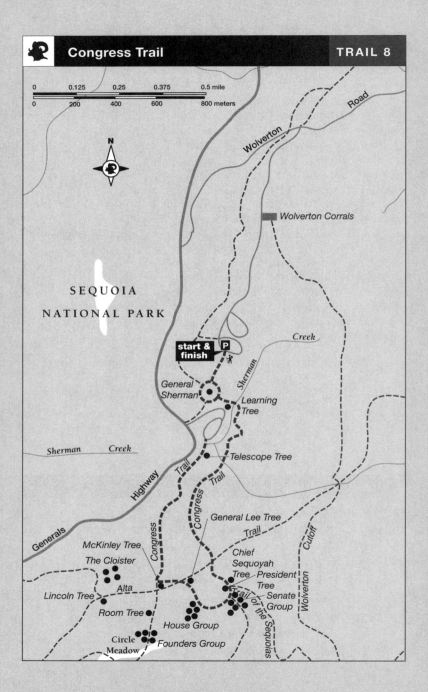

Congress Trail

TRAIL 8

| 0 | 0.125 | 0.25 | 0.375 | 0.5 mile |
| 0 | 200 | 400 | 600 | 800 meters |

N

Road

Wolverton

Wolverton Corrals

SEQUOIA

NATIONAL PARK

Creek

start & finish   P

General Sherman

Sherman

Learning Tree

Sherman   Creek

Telescope Tree

Highway

Trail

Congress   Trail

General Lee Tree

Generals

Trail

Cutoff

McKinley Tree

The Cloister

Congress

Chief Sequoyah Tree   President Tree

Senate Group

Wolverton

Lincoln Tree

Alta

Trail of the Sequoias

Room Tree

House Group

Circle Meadow

Founders Group

Congress Trail

Not surprisingly, the largest tree in the world is an attraction guaranteed to lure throngs of tourists, both domestic and international, throughout the course of a Sierra summer. With the General Sherman Tree as the first stop, this 3-plus-mile, paved loop also visits the fourth, fifth, and 29th largest giant sequoias, and two of the most impressive clusters of the big trees, the Senate and House groups. Short side trips offer even more possibilities for viewing other notable Giant Forest landmarks. While you shouldn't expect to stand alone in reverent solitude before these awe-inspiring monarchs of the forest, the numbers of tourists drops dramatically the farther you travel away from the General Sherman Tree.

Best Times

Snow generally leaves the trails sometime in May in this part of the Giant Forest, permitting snow-free hiking until the first winter storm, usually in late October or early November. Late spring, when the azalea flowers are in bloom, is a particularly fine time for a visit, as is early fall, when the azalea leaves are cloaked in autumn splendor. Colorful wildflowers put on a showy display in early summer.

Finding the Trail

From Visalia, follow Highway 198 to Three Rivers and proceed east into Sequoia National Park, where the road becomes Generals Highway. Follow Generals Highway to the Giant Forest. The parking

TRAIL USE
Dayhike, Child Friendly
LENGTH
3.1 miles, 1½–2 hours
VERTICAL FEET
+550/-550/±1100
DIFFICULTY
– 1 **2** 3 4 5 +
TRAIL TYPE
Loop

FEATURES
Fall Colors
Wildflowers
Giant Sequoias

FACILITIES
Restrooms
Water
Shuttle Bus Stop

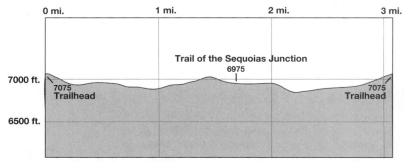

TRAIL 8 Congress Trail Elevation Profile

area for the General Sherman Tree (and start of the Congress Trail) was relocated in 2005 to provide a less environmentally sensitive site than the previous one just off the Generals Highway. Visitors can opt for riding the free shuttle bus from the Giant Forest Museum to the old parking area near the General Sherman Tree (saving a little less than a mile of walking), or for driving their vehicle on the Generals Highway to the Wolverton Road, 1.75 miles south of Lodgepole and 2.8 miles north of the museum. Motorists should then follow the Wolverton Road 0.5 mile to a three-way stop and then turn right to follow a spur road another half mile to the General Sherman parking area at the end of the road. Lodgepole is the nearest campground (fee, flush toilets, running water, bear boxes, phone). Wuksachi Village, a short distance north of Lodgepole, offers upscale lodging and dining.

> The diameter of the tree's largest branch is an amazing 7 feet, larger than the diameter of the trunk on most mature conifers.

Trail Description

▶1 From the parking lot, pass through an elaborate wood archway lined with informational placards and descend along a well-graded, paved trail with periodic stairs toward the General Sherman Tree. Several park benches along the way offer tourists convenient resting spots for the uphill return. Where the path makes a sharp bend, a set of stairs marks the beginning of the lightly used Lodgepole and Sherman Tree Trail that connects these two areas. Farther on, a wide spot in the trail is imprinted with a cross section of the Sherman Tree's base, a graphic picture of this truly massive giant sequoia. This spot also offers an unobstructed view of the world's largest tree, distant enough for photographers to squeeze the big tree into their camera frames. A short walk beyond the vista leads to a junction of the nature trail to **General Sherman** on the right and the signed **Congress Trail** on the left.

 Giant Sequoias

Whether you arrive via the shuttle bus or by way of the half-mile trail from the parking area, find the signed trailhead for the **Congress Trail** nearby ►2 and proceed downhill to the Leaning Tree. From there, the path continues over a pair of footbridges over branches of Sherman Creek, passing a number of stately sequoias along the way. Springtime hikers will notice the lovely white blooms of dogwoods scattered throughout the Giant Forest, while autumn hikers will be blessed by the fall colors from the turning leaves. Beyond the second bridge, a lateral on the right ►3 offers a shortcut back to

 Fall Colors

General Sherman Tree

NOTE

Any visit to the Giant Forest would be incomplete without taking the short stroll around this immense monarch of the forest. At 275 feet high, 103 feet around the base, and with a volume of 52,508 cubic feet, this giant sequoia has been declared not only the world's biggest tree but also the largest living organism in existence. The diameter of the tree's largest branch is an amazing 7 feet, larger than the diameter of the trunk on most mature conifers. James Wolverton, a pioneer cattleman who served under the general during the Civil War, named the tree in 1879 for General William Tecumseh Sherman, whose most remembered act during the war was the dubious March to the Sea, a campaign across Georgia from Atlanta.

the trailhead for those unaccustomed to hiking at 7000 feet.

From the lateral, a winding, quarter-mile ascent leads to a four-way junction with the Alta Trail. ▶4 Beyond the junction, nearing the south end of the loop, are many notable sequoias, including Chief Sequoyah (29th largest) and the President (fourth

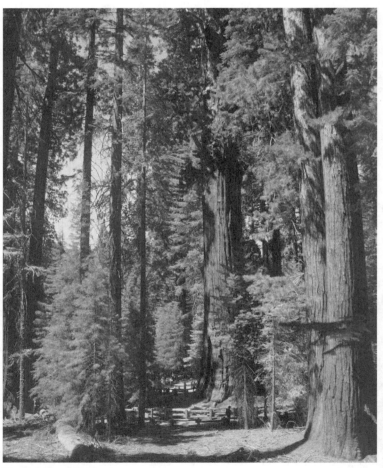

General Sherman Tree

largest), the Senate and House groups, and General Lee and McKinley trees. Amid the staid **Senate Group**, the Trail of the Sequoias branches south. ▶5 After 0.3 mile, reach a five-way junction with the Alta and Circle Meadows trails near the McKinley Tree. ▶6 With extra time, you can visit additional sequoia landmarks on easy side trips from this junction. The Cloister Tree and Lincoln Tree (fifth largest) are just a short jaunt southwest on the Alta Trail. A longer, 0.9-mile excursion farther southwest on the Alta Trail leads to the **Huckleberry Meadow Trail** and a short walk generally south to the Washington Tree (second largest). Southbound, the Circle Meadow Trail takes you shortly to the Room Tree, the Founders Group, and Cattle Cabin.

From the five-way junction, head north to descend mildly on the **Congress Trail**, weaving through the forest back to the lateral shortcut. ▶7 From there, continue north to the vicinity of the General Sherman Tree ▶8, and either pick up the shuttle bus or retrace your steps uphill to the parking area. ▶9

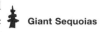

Giant Sequoias

🚶	**MILESTONES**	
▶1	0.0	Start at General Sherman parking area
▶2	0.4	General Sherman Nature Trail and trailhead for Congress Trail
▶3	0.8	Straight at lateral junction
▶4	1.2	Straight at Alta Trail junction
▶5	1.7	Veer right at Trail of the Sequoias junction
▶6	2.0	Turn right (north) at five-way junction with Alta and Circle Meadow trails
▶7	2.4	Straight at lateral junction
▶8	2.7	General Sherman Tree and trailhead for Congress Trail
▶9	3.1	Parking area

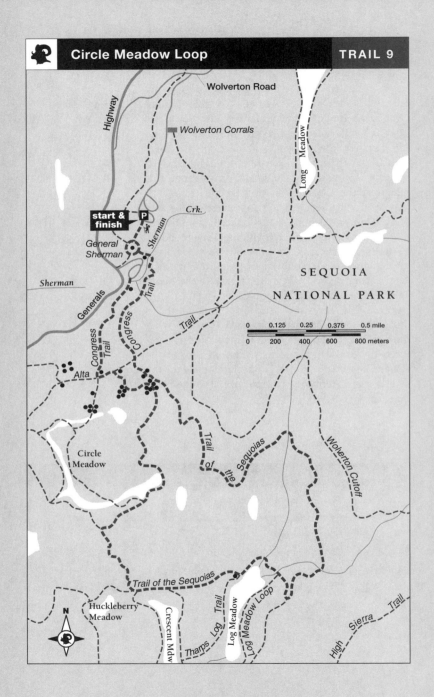

Circle Meadow Loop

TRAIL 9

Wolverton Road

Wolverton Corrals

Highway

Long Meadow

Crk.

start & finish

P

Sherman

General Sherman

Sherman

Sherman Trail

Generals

Congress Trail

Trail

SEQUOIA

NATIONAL PARK

| 0 | 0.125 | 0.25 | 0.375 | 0.5 mile |

| 0 | 200 | 400 | 600 | 800 meters |

Alta

Congress Trail

Circle Meadow

Trail of the Sequoias

Wolverton Cutoff

Trail of the Sequoias

Huckleberry Meadow

N

Crescent Mdw

Tharps Log Trail

Log Meadow

Log Meadow Loop

High Sierra Trail

Circle Meadow Loop

This trip provides dayhikers with a journey of contrasts. Beginning and ending on the heavily used Congress Trail, the middle part of the loop breaks away from the popular path for a venture farther into the heart of Giant Forest, where visitors should be able to enjoy a more serene encounter with some of the monarchs of the forest. Along with the popular Giant Forest landmarks of the General Sherman, Learning, and Chief Sequoyah trees, this loop visits such attractions as Black Arch, Pillars of Hercules, Cattle Cabin, Founders Group, and the Room Tree. In addition, verdant Circle Meadow will delight visitors with a slender, flower-filled clearing rimmed by statuesque trees.

Best Times

Snow generally leaves the trails sometime in May in this part of Giant Forest, permitting snow-free hiking until the first winter storm, usually in late October or early November. Late spring, when the azalea flowers are in bloom, is a particularly fine time for a visit, as is early fall, when the azalea leaves are cloaked in autumn splendor. Colorful wildflowers put on a showy display in early summer.

Finding the Trail

From Visalia, follow Highway 198 to Three Rivers and proceed east into Sequoia National Park, where the road becomes Generals Highway. Follow Generals Highway to Giant Forest. The parking area for the General Sherman Tree (and start of the Congress

TRAIL USE
Dayhike, Child Friendly
LENGTH
5.8 miles, 3 hours
VERTICAL FEET
+850/-850/±1700
DIFFICULTY
– 1 **2** 3 4 5 +
TRAIL TYPE
Loop

FEATURES
Fall Colors
Wildflowers
Giant Sequoias
Secluded

FACILITIES
Restrooms
Water
Shuttle Bus Stop

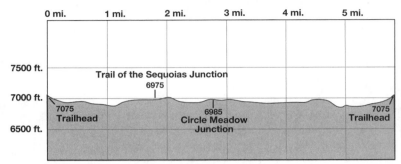

| 0 mi. | 1 mi. | 2 mi. | 3 mi. | 4 mi. | 5 mi. |

7500 ft.

Trail of the Sequoias Junction
6975

7000 ft.

7075
Trailhead

6985
Circle Meadow
Junction

7075
Trailhead

6500 ft.

TRAIL 9 Circle Meadow Loop Elevation Profile

Trail) was relocated in 2005 to provide a less environmentally sensitive site than the previous one just off the Generals Highway. Visitors can opt for riding the free shuttle bus from the Giant Forest Museum to the old parking area near the General Sherman Tree (saving a mile of walking), or for driving their vehicle on the Generals Highway to the Wolverton Road, 1.75 miles south of Lodgepole and 2.8 miles north of the museum. Motorists should then follow the Wolverton Road to the right-hand turn for the spur road to the General Sherman parking area and continue to the end of the road. Lodgepole is the nearest campground (fee, flush toilets, running water, bear boxes, phone). Wuksachi Village, a short distance north of Lodgepole, offers upscale lodging and dining.

Trail Description

►1 From the parking lot, descend along a well-graded trail for a half mile to the **General Sherman Tree**, at 275 feet high, 103 feet around at the base, and with a volume of 52,508 cubic feet, the largest giant sequoia in the world.

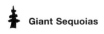

Giant Sequoias

Whether you arrived via the shuttle bus, or by way of the half-mile trail from the parking area, find the signed trailhead for the Congress Trail nearby

▶**2** and proceed downhill to the Leaning Tree. From there, the path continues over a pair of footbridges over branches of Sherman Creek, passing by a number of stately sequoias along the way. Beyond the second bridge, a lateral on the right ▶**3** offers a shortcut back to the trailhead for those unaccustomed to hiking at 7000 feet.

From the lateral, a winding, quarter-mile ascent leads to a four-way junction with the Alta Trail. ▶**4** Beyond the junction, nearing the south end of the loop, are many notable sequoias, including Chief Sequoyah (29th largest) and the President (fourth largest), the Senate and House groups, and General Lee and McKinley trees. Amid the staid **Senate Group**, turn left and follow the **Trail of the Sequoias** branching south. ▶**5**

Proceed through the mature sequoias of the Senate Group and then follow a gentle descent past a couple of scorched giants that at first glance appear dead, but after further inspection you can see that they are, amazingly, still alive. Cross a tiny rivulet trickling into the east end of lush Circle Meadow and then follow the path across a hillside above the edge of this verdant clearing. Pass the unsigned fork of a use trail heading out into the meadow and reach a junction with the designated **Circle Meadow Trail** a short distance farther. ▶**6**

Turn right and immediately cross the thin ribbon of Circle Meadow. Beyond the meadow, you climb a low hill and reach Black Arch, another interesting scorched giant, and then Pillars of Hercules, where the trail passes right between two massive sequoias. Proceed along the western fringe of Circle Meadow, passing a junction ▶**7** with a little-used trail heading northwest on the way to **Cattle Cabin.** This structure was built by cattlemen who pastured their stock in the meadows nearby. Just beyond the cabin, step across another tiny rivulet that courses through the northern swath of the meadow and then continue

Verdant Circle Meadow will delight visitors with a slender, flower-filled clearing rimmed by statuesque trees.

through the **Founders Group**, a stand of a dozen stately sequoias named in honor of the citizens who assisted in the establishment of Sequoia National Park. Not far from the Founders Group is the **Room Tree**, a giant sequoia with a small passageway in the trunk that leads into a large, hollowed-out section at the base of the tree. A short way farther is a five-way junction between the Circle Meadow, Alta, and Congress trails. ▶8

From the five-way junction, head north to descend mildly on the Congress Trail, weaving through the forest back to the lateral shortcut. ▶9 From there, continue north to the vicinity of the **General Sherman Tree** ▶10, and either pick up the shuttle bus or retrace your steps uphill to the parking area. ▶11

🚶	**MILESTONES**	
▶1	0.0	Start at General Sherman parking area
▶2	0.5	General Sherman Nature Trail and trailhead for Congress Trail
▶3	0.9	Straight at lateral junction
▶4	1.3	Straight at Alta Trail junction
▶5	1.8	Turn left (south) at Trail of the Sequoias junction
▶6	2.8	Turn right (northwest) at Circle Meadow junction
▶7	3.3	Straight at connector
▶8	3.6	Straight (north) at Congress and Alta trails junction
▶9	4.0	Straight at lateral junction
▶10	4.3	General Sherman Tree and trailhead for Congress Trail
▶11	5.8	Parking area

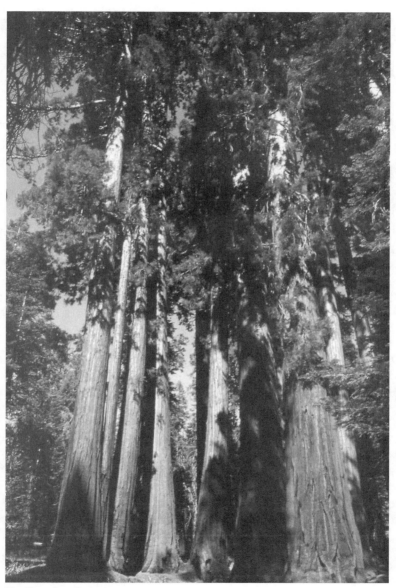

The Founders Group

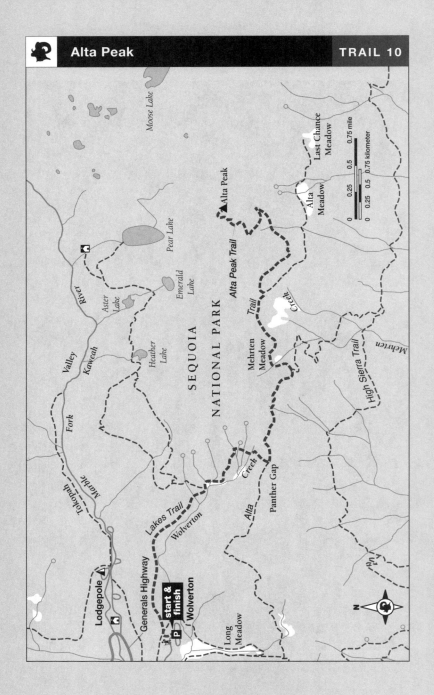

Moose Lake

Last Chance Meadow

0.75 mile

0.5

0.25

0.75 kilometer

0.5

0.25

0

▲Alta Peak

Alta Meadow

Pear Lake

Alta Peak Trail

Emerald Lake

Mehrten Trail

Creek

Aster Lake

River

SEQUOIA

NATIONAL PARK

Mehrten Meadow

Heather Lake

Valley

High Sierra Trail

Kaweah

Fork

Creek

Alta

Panther Gap

Marble

Tokopah

Lakes Trail

Wolverton

Generals Highway

Lodgepole

start & finish

P

Wolverton

Long Meadow

N

Alta Peak

Alta Peak's airy summit offers one of the best views available on the western side of Sequoia via a maintained trail. While arduous, a one-day ascent is a viable option for strong hikers who are well acclimatized. Lesser mortals have the option of a 2–3 day backpack trip, with a basecamp at either Alta Meadow or Mehrten Meadow Camp. However many days are needed, the supreme vista from Alta Peak is a just reward for the effort involved in getting there.

Best Time

The trail to Alta Peak, with a summit elevation of more than 11,000 feet, is usually snowbound through early July. The most popular time to climb the peak is midsummer, when there is the bonus of a fine wildflower display along the way. Early autumn is still a good time for an ascent, although hikers must be prepared for chilly temperatures. Once the first significant snowfall hits the southern Sierra, generally by the end of October, the trail holds onto snow until next summer.

Finding the Trail

From Visalia, follow Highway 198 to Three Rivers and proceed east into Sequoia National Park, where the road becomes Generals Highway. Follow Generals Highway to the Wolverton Road, 1.75 miles southeast of Lodgepole. Head east for 1.5 miles on Wolverton Road to the large trailhead parking area. Lodgepole is the nearest campground

TRAIL USE
Dayhike, Backpack, Horse

LENGTH
13.4 miles, 7–8 hours

VERTICAL FEET
+4275/-350/±9250

DIFFICULTY
– 1 2 3 4 **5** +

TRAIL TYPE
Out & Back

FEATURES
Mountain
Summit
Wildflowers
Great Views
Camping
Steep

FACILITIES
Restrooms
Water
Bear Boxes

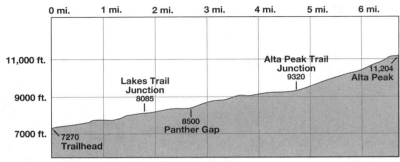

TRAIL 10 Alta Peak Elevation Profile

(fee, flush toilets, running water, bear boxes, and phone). Wuksachi Village, a short distance north of Lodgepole, offers upscale lodging and dining.

Logistics

Backpackers must obtain a wilderness permit for all overnight visits. See page 28 for more details about how to obtain one.

Trail Description

▶1 A barrage of trail signs with numerous destinations and mileages marks the start of the trail. Follow a series of concrete steps shortly to a wide, single-track dirt trail that ascends a hillside to a junction at the crest with a path accessing the Lodgepole area and the Wolverton corrals. ▶2 Turn right and follow the **Lakes Trail**, soon passing another junction with a trail on the right to Long Meadow. ▶3 After the initial ascent, the grade eases to more of a mild to moderate climb along the course of Wolverton Creek. Hop across a spring-fed tributary of the creek and proceed to a junction with the trail to Panther Gap. ▶4

Turn right and follow well-maintained tread through moderate forest cover on a course that roughly parallels **Wolverton Creek**, stepping across numerous little tributary streams along the way. Eventually, these delightful brooks lined with lush foliage are left behind, as the trail climbs out of the canyon to a T-junction with the **Alta Trail** at Panther Gap. ►5

Heading east on the Alta Trail, the trail soon veers onto the open, south-facing slope above Middle Fork Kaweah River, where views across this deep cleft are quite impressive. After a half mile, you hop across a nascent tributary of Panther Creek and then follow a series of switchbacks to a junction with the Sevenmile Trail. ►6 Remaining on the Alta Trail, proceed into forest cover and down to a ford of Mehrten Creek. Nearby is **Mehrten Meadow Camp**, ►7 where a few campsites with a bear box are sheltered by red firs. The narrow glade of Mehrten Meadow lies well below the trail. Leaving Mehrten Creek behind, the trail follows a mildly ascending, ¾-mile traverse across the north wall of the canyon to a junction with the **Alta Peak Trail**. ►8

You turn left and zigzag up the hillside beneath the intermittent shade from a grove of red firs, before

 Great Views

 Camping

OPTIONS

Alta Meadow

Overnighters may find favorable campsites near Alta Meadow. From the junction of Alta and Alta Peak trails, follow mildly ascending trail around the forested base of Tharps Rock, eventually breaking out of the trees to a wide-ranging view of Middle Fork Kaweah River canyon. Beyond a stream crossing, the trail reaches the northwestern fringe of the verdant and flower-covered meadowlands of **Alta Meadow,** the beauty of which is complemented exquisitely by views of Tharps Rock, Alta Peak, and the Kings-Kaweah and Great Western divides. Fine campsites are nestled beneath red firs on a low ridge just south of the trail. An unmaintained path continues a short distance east over vales and rivulets to Last Chance Meadow and additional campsites.

the trees are soon left behind on an ascent to a refreshing, spring-fed, willow- and wildflower-lined stream. Ford the stream, pass a small campsite near the east bank, and begin a long ascending traverse across the face of Tharps Rock through scattered red firs and patches of chinquapin. Excellent views abound across the deep canyon of Middle Fork Kaweah River to the terrain in the southwestern part of Sequoia National Park, as well as the verdant swath of Alta Meadow below, and Tharps Rock and Alta Peak above. Nearing the end of the traverse, you reach the last reliable water source at a pretty arroyo filled with heather and wildflowers.

Following a switchback, the trail climbs stiffly on a zigzagging course above Tharps Rock. A few stunted foxtail pines herald the arrival into the alpine zone, where scattered tufts of ground-

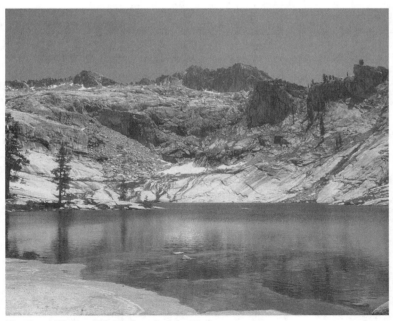

The Great Western Divide *from the Lakes Trail*

hugging flowers and plants cling to the nearly barren slopes. Over decomposed granite and around boulders, the unrelenting ascent continues just below the southwest ridge to the crest of the summit ridge. A short climb from there leads to the summit block and a final scramble to the top of **Alta Peak**. ►9

To describe the view from the summit as spectacular is an understatement. The body of water directly north of the peak is Pear Lake, backdropped by a sea of granite rising northeast to the Tableland and the **Kings-Kaweah Divide**. Numerous park landmarks are clearly visible, including the **Sierra Crest** stretching across the eastern horizon. With the aid of a big enough map, you'll be able to identify scads of peaks. When the ubiquitous San Joaquin Valley haze is absent, usually only after a rare, cleansing summer rainstorm, you'll be blessed with a western view across the valley's farmland to the Coast Range.

 Summit

 Great Views

🚶	**MILESTONES**	
►1	0.0	Start at trailhead
►2	0.1	Turn right (east) at junction
►3	0.15	Straight at junction to Long Meadow
►4	1.8	Veer right (south) at junction to Panther Gap
►5	2.7	Turn left at Alta Trail junction
►6	3.2	Straight at Sevenmile Trail junction
►7	4.0	Mehrten Meadow Camp
►8	4.75	Veer left (north) at Alta Peak Trail junction
►9	6.7	Alta Peak

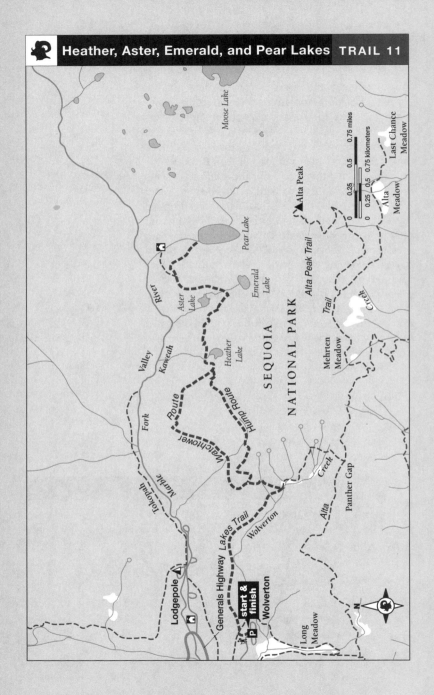

Moose Lake

Pear Lake

Emerald Lake

Aster Lake

Heather Lake

SEQUOIA

NATIONAL PARK

Alta Peak

Alta Peak Trail

Mehrten Meadow Trail

Creek

Alta Meadow

Last Chance Meadow

River

Valley

Kaweah

Fork

Marble

Tokopah

Watchtower Route

Hump Route

Generals Highway

Lakes Trail

Wolverton

Alta Creek

Panther Gap

Lodgepole

start & finish

P Wolverton

Long Meadow

N

0 0.25 0.5 0.75 miles
0 0.25 0.5 0.75 kilometers

Heather, Aster, Emerald, and Pear Lakes

The Lakes Trail to Heather, Aster, Emerald, and Pear lakes is one of the busiest trails in Sequoia National Park, thanks to a combination of spectacular scenery and easy access. All four lakes are quite picturesque and provide fine opportunities for sunbathing on granite slabs around the shore, or for taking a refreshing afternoon dip in the chilly waters. Anglers can try their luck on the resident trout as well. In addition to the lovely lakes, plenty of dramatic vistas can be had along the way, including an incredible view of Tokopah Valley and the tumbling Marble Fork Kaweah River from the Watchtower Route, which follows a narrow ledge across a sheer face dynamited out of the rock some 2000 feet above the valley floor. An early start should allow hikers in good condition to complete the trip in about 12 hours.

Due to the lakes' popularity, the Park Service has instituted camping bans at Heather and Aster lakes, and limited camping to designated sites near Emerald and Pear lakes. In addition, visitors are encouraged to use the backcountry pit toilets placed in the vicinity of the lakes. With a basecamp at Pear Lake, the open granite terrain to the east is well suited for cross-country travel to Moose Lake and the Tableland. Equestrians are limited to day-use trips.

Best Time

The Lakes Trail usually sheds its snow by mid-June, with wildflower season beginning in earnest by early July. The trail is busy with dayhikers from then

TRAIL USE
Dayhike, Backpack, Horse

LENGTH
11.5 miles, 6–7 hours

VERTICAL FEET
+2800/-550/±6700

DIFFICULTY
– 1 2 3 **4** 5 +

TRAIL TYPE
Out & Back

FEATURES
Mountain
Lake
Wildflowers
Great Views
Camping
Swimming

FACILITIES
Restrooms
Water
Bear Boxes

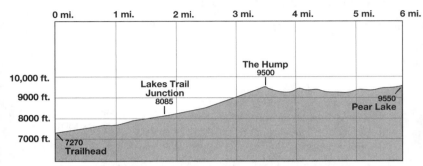

TRAIL 11 Heather, Aster, Emerald, and Pear Lakes Elevation Profile

Emerald Lake, backdropped by steep cliffs on three sides, is picturesquely set below Alta Peak.

through Labor Day weekend, when backcountry permits are also at a premium. The crowds disperse considerably after Labor Day, making September a fine time for either a dayhike or backpack.

Finding the Trail

From Visalia, follow Highway 198 to Three Rivers and proceed east into Sequoia National Park, where the road becomes Generals Highway. Follow Generals Highway to the Wolverton Road, 1.75 miles southeast of Lodgepole. Head east for 1.5 miles on Wolverton Road to the large trailhead parking area. Lodgepole is the nearest campground (fee, flush toilets, running water, bear boxes, and phone). Wuksachi Village, a short distance north of Lodgepole, offers upscale lodging and dining.

Logistics

Backpackers must obtain a wilderness permit for all overnight visits. See page 28 for more details about how to obtain one.

Trail Description

▶1 A barrage of trail signs with numerous destinations and mileages marks the start of the trail. Follow a series of concrete steps shortly to a wide, single-track dirt trail that ascends a hillside to a junction at the crest with a path accessing the Lodgepole area and the Wolverton corrals. ▶2 Turn right and follow the **Lakes Trail**, soon passing another junction with a trail on the right to Long Meadow. ▶3 After the initial ascent, the grade eases to more of a mild to moderate climb along the course of Wolverton Creek. Hop across a spring-fed tributary of the creek and proceed to a junction with the trail to Panther Gap. ▶4

Remaining on the Lakes Trail, turn left at the junction, weave up a hillside, and then drop briefly to the crossing of a flower- and fern-lined **tributary of Wolverton Creek**. A moderate climb ensues on the way to a junction ▶5 between the Watchtower Route on the left and the Hump Route on the right.

 Wildflowers

Turn right and follow switchbacks on a moderate to moderately steep climb through red fir forest, crossing a tiny stream lined with pockets of flower-dotted meadow along the way. At the apex of the climb you gain the crest of **the Hump**, ▶6 where a splendid vista of the Tableland and Silliman Crest can be had by stepping off the trail toward an open stretch of hillside beyond scattered conifers.

A steep descent leads down to a small flat, carpeted with pockets of heather and dotted with a smattering of lodgepole pines, where the two routes

 Cross-Country Options

Even though the maintained trail ends at Pear Lake, experienced cross-country enthusiasts can venture further afield on off-trail excursions to remote **Moose Lake** and the **Tableland**.

Return via the Watchtower

For a scenic variation on your return to the trailhead, retrace your steps back to the junction ►7 between the Watchtower and the Hump routes, 0.2 mile west of Heather Lake. Bear right at the junction and follow the **Watchtower Route** on a gentle descent. Soon the trail starts clinging to the side of a near-vertical cliff that plunges 2000 feet straight down to Tokopah Valley. Not surprisingly, the exposed view down to the churning and careening Marble Fork is quite staggering (severe acrophobes will be best served by avoiding this route altogether and returning to the trailhead via the Hump Route). The thunderous sound of the river reverberates all the way up to the level of the trail. With all of the drama below, don't forget to turn around and experience the vista of the **Silliman Crest**.

Proceed down the trail on a moderate descent that leads to a wedge of rock protruding into the canyon, shown as Point 8973T on the USGS 7.5-minute *Lodgepole* quadrangle. An unofficial scramble route leads bold adventurers to extraordinary views from the top of this feature. Beyond the wedge of rock, switchbacks head down less precipitous slopes and into light forest cover. Hop over a vigorous creek lined with lush foliage and continue descending moderately to the junction where the Hump and Watchtower routes come together again. ►5 From there, retrace your steps 2.1 miles to the trailhead. ►1

merge at a signed junction. ►7 From the junction, a brief, mild descent offers a glimpse of **Heather Lake** below, near where a lateral leads shortly to a pit toilet; the facility is screened on three sides, which allows for a splendid view. Just beyond the lateral, you reach the heather-laced shore of aptly named Heather Lake, ►8 where a few pines formerly sheltered a number of campsites around the cliff-rimmed shoreline, but the area has been closed to camping for several years due to overuse.

 Lake

Proceed on rocky tread around boulders and scattered pines on a climb out of the Heather Lake basin. Once out of the basin, the trail leads across open granite terrain on a gentler grade, with fine

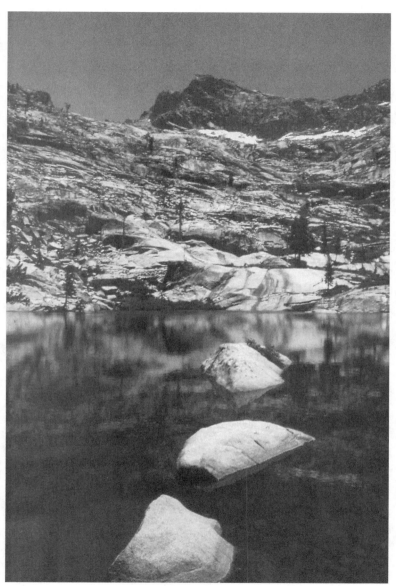

Emerald Lake

views across the canyon of Marble Fork Kaweah River and up to Alta Peak. Wrap around a hillside and then drop to the floor of a basin cradling **Aster Lake**, 0.2 mile downhill to the left, and **Emerald Lake**, a shorter distance uphill to the right. ►9 Although camping is banned at Aster Lake, granite slabs around the mostly open shoreline afford fine spots for sunbathing. Anglers can test their skills on the resident rainbow trout. Between the trail and Emerald Lake, designated campsites with bear boxes offer backpackers the first opportunity for legal camping between here and the trailhead. Scattered pines shelter the campsites and thin strips of verdant meadow border the nearby outlet. Emerald Lake, backdropped by steep cliffs on three sides, is picturesquely set below Alta Peak. Above the far shore, the inlet cascades dramatically down cliffs before gracefully pouring across granite slabs on the way into the lake. Brook trout will tempt the angler at Emerald Lake. Between the two lakes is a solar toilet.

A mildly ascending trail leads away from the Emerald and Aster lakes basin around a spur ridge and into the Pear Lake basin, where small pockets of wildflowers soften the otherwise rocky terrain. Fine views into the deep cleft of Marble Fork Kaweah River and Tokopah Valley capture your attention as you follow the trail around the spur. Pass a junction with a trail on the left to the Pear Lake ranger station and continue on ascending tread for another half mile to rockbound **Pear Lake**. ►10 Rimmed by craggy ridges and towered over by Alta Peak, the lake is quite scenic, with widely scattered pines and small tufts of grass finding tenuous footholds in the stony basin. Campers will find 12 designated campsites spread around the outlet, with a solar toilet nearby. Anglers can fish for brook trout.

 Lake

 Fishing

 Camping

 Great Views

🚶 MILESTONES

►1   0.0   Start at trailhead

►2   0.1   Turn right (east) at junction

►3   0.15   Straight at junction to Long Meadow

►4   1.8   Veer left (south) at junction to Panther Gap

►5   2.1   Turn right (east) at first Watchtower/Hump junction

►6   3.4   The Hump

►7   3.6   Straight at second Watchtower/Hump junction

►8   3.8   Heather Lake

►9   4.7   Aster and Emerald lakes

►10 5.75   Pear Lake

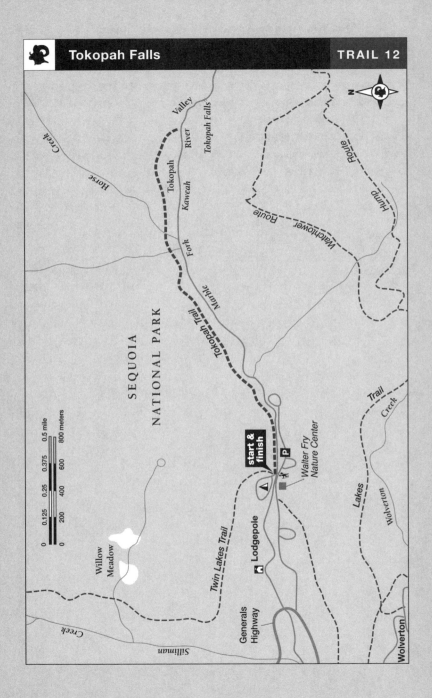

Tokopah Falls

TRAIL 12

N

Horse Creek

Tokopah Valley

Kaweah River

Tokopah Falls

Hump Route

Watchtower Route

Tokopah

Kaweah

Fork

Marble

Tokopah Trail

SEQUOIA
NATIONAL PARK

Trail

Creek

start & finish

P

Walter Fry
Nature Center

Twin Lakes Trail

Lakes

Wolverton

Willow
Meadow

Lodgepole

0   0.125   0.25   0.375   0.5 mile

0   200   400   600   800 meters

Generals
Highway

Silliman Creek

Wolverton

Tokopah Falls

An easy 2-mile hike leads to a viewpoint of Tokopah Falls, where the waters from Marble Fork Kaweah River plunge down a steep headwall at the upper end of Tokopah Valley. While the falls are best viewed in late spring, the straightforward hike is also quite pleasant in summer and fall. The nearby amenities at Lodgepole Village offer plenty of extra diversions.

Best Time

Tokopah Valley is usually snow-free from April to November. However, the falls are in full glory when snowmelt in the higher elevations turns Marble Fork Kaweah River into a raging torrent during late spring and early summer.

Finding the Trail

From Visalia, follow Highway 198 to Three Rivers and proceed east into Sequoia National Park, where the road becomes Generals Highway. Drive on Generals Highway to the Lodgepole junction and turn east. Proceed to the entrance station for Lodgepole Campground (fee, flush toilets, running water, bear boxes, and phone) to secure a free parking permit and then continue to the hiker and backpacker parking area. Wuksachi Village, a short distance north of Lodgepole, offers upscale lodging and dining.

TRAIL USE
Dayhike, Horse

LENGTH
4.1 miles, 2 hours

VERTICAL FEET
+700/±1400

DIFFICULTY
− 1 **2** 3 4 5 +

TRAIL TYPE
Out & Back

FEATURES
Canyon
Waterfall
Wildflowers
Great Views

FACILITIES
Store
Visitors Center
Nature Center
Post Office
Campground
Picnic Area
Restrooms
Laundromat
Showers
Phone
Water
Bear Boxes
Shuttle Bus Stop

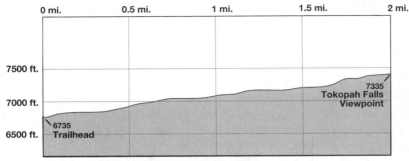

TRAIL 12 Tokopah Falls Elevation Profile

Trail Description

Early in the year the roar of the falls can be quite deafening, as a snowmelt-filled torrent catapults over the lip of the canyon headwall.

►1 From the parking area, walk along the campground access road past the Walter Fry Nature Center and restrooms to a fork in the road ►2 and veer left. Cross a log bridge over the Marble Fork and locate the beginning of the **Tokopah Trail** on the far side. ►3 Head upstream from the trailhead on single-track trail on a mild climb through a mixed forest of red and white firs, incense cedars, and ponderosa and Jeffrey pines, with the river lined by willows, aspens, and chokecherrys. Proceed up the north bank, sometimes right alongside the churning river and sometimes a fair distance away. Low granite outcrops and small pockets of grassy meadow sprinkled with early season wildflowers break up the otherwise continuous band of trees. Several short bridges span seasonal swales on the way up Tokopah Valley.

Depending on the time of year, you may hear Tokopah Falls well before you actually see the sometimes-mighty cascade. Early in the year the roar of the falls can be quite deafening, as a snowmelt-filled torrent catapults over the lip of the canyon headwall. Eventually, the forest gives way to shrubs of elderberry, oak, and manzanita growing between piles of boulders and large blocks of granite, finally allowing views of the falls and the steep-walled canyon.

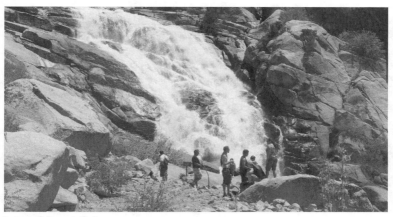

Lower Tokopah Falls

Across the canyon looms the mighty wall of rock known as **the Watchtower**, which soars 2000 feet above the valley floor. **Canyon**

The trail continues ascending through a sea of boulders and slabs, increasing in grade on the approach to the base of the falls. The trail abruptly terminates ►4 at a boulder-rimmed bench near the base of some steep cliffs, where a sign advises against the idea of attempting further progress up the canyon onto slippery and unstable slopes (some fatalities have occurred here over the years). Ahead, silvery **Tokopah Falls** creates a majestic scene, plummeting down the steep headwall of the upper canyon. Once you've fully enjoyed the falls, retrace your steps to the trailhead.

Waterfall

🚶	**MILESTONES**	
►1	0.0	Start at parking area
►2	0.1	Veer left at fork in the road
►3	0.15	Start of Tokopah Trail
►4	2.05	End of trail

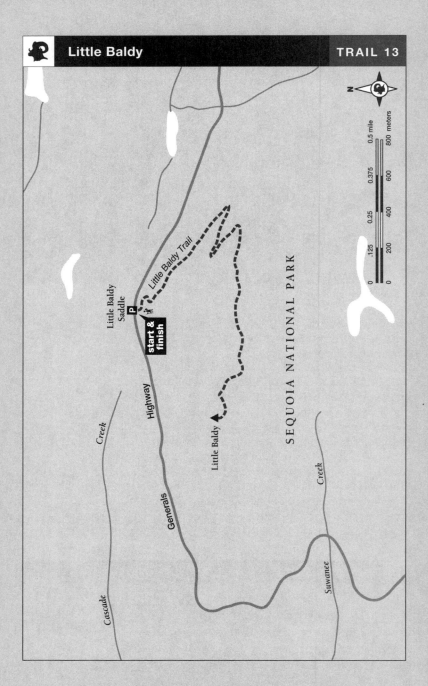

Little Baldy

TRAIL 13

N

0 .125 0.25 0.375 0.5 mile
0 200 400 600 800 meters

Little Baldy Trail

Little Baldy Saddle

start & finish

Highway

Little Baldy

SEQUOIA NATIONAL PARK

Creek

Generals

Cascade

Creek

Suwanee

Little Baldy

An excellent vista gained by a less than 2-mile hike should tempt just about any self-respecting hiker. A moderate climb of 700-plus feet leads to arguably one of the western Sierra's supreme views from the top of Little Baldy, a vista so expansive that the Park Service used to maintain a fire lookout there. Reach the trailhead with plenty of water, as none is readily available en route or anywhere nearby. Despite the lack of water, a few parties each year spend a night on the summit, undoubtedly drawn by the incomparable sunsets and excellent stargazing.

Best Time

The absolute best time to enjoy the view from the top of Little Baldy is following a rare cleansing storm, when the rains have washed the ubiquitous haze from the skies above the San Joaquin Valley. Thankfully, the eastward view of the Great Western Divide and other notable features in the park is not as dependent on the air quality above the valley, making a snow-free hike anytime from June to mid-October a rewarding experience.

Finding the Trail

From Visalia, follow Highway 198 to Three Rivers and proceed east into Sequoia National Park, where the road becomes Generals Highway. Follow Generals Highway to Little Baldy Saddle, 6.6 miles north of the Lodgepole turnoff (17 miles south of the Y-junction with Highway 180). Park your vehicle along the shoulder as space allows. Dorst

TRAIL USE
Dayhike

LENGTH
3.5 miles, 2 hours

VERTICAL FEET
+750/-75/±1650

DIFFICULTY
– 1 2 **3** 4 5 +

TRAIL TYPE
Out & Back

FEATURES
Mountain
Summit
Great Views

FACILITIES
None

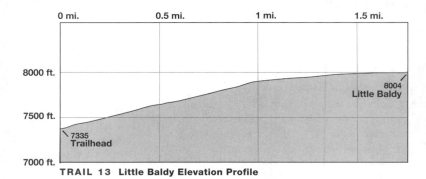

TRAIL 13 Little Baldy Elevation Profile

Campground (fee, flush toilets, running water, bear boxes, and phone) is the nearest campground. Wuksachi Village, a short distance north of Lodgepole, offers upscale lodging and dining. Stony Creek Village and Montecito Lake Resort offer slightly less expensive lodging options.

Trail Description

▶1 From the roadside trail sign, head up the trail on a climb of a hillside covered with red firs and a smattering of Jeffrey pines. Beyond a pair of switchbacks, the trail makes a steady, moderate climb northeast across a steep hillside, roughly paralleling the highway below. Sporadic gaps in the forest allow brief views of Big Baldy to the northwest, while the craggy spires of Chimney Rock can be seen directly ahead. After a trio of switchbacks, the grade eases along the ridge north of **Little Baldy,** as you proceed toward the summit through pockets of forest, manzanita, and oak. A final short and rocky climb leads to the top and the extraordinary view. ▶2

▲ Summit

From the summit, the view encompasses a large part of the **Great Western Divide,** as well as features closer at hand, such as Castle Rocks and Mineral King valley to the southeast. To the southwest is a rugged and remote section of Sequoia

🔭 Great Views

National Park, where a once prominent network of trails has mostly disappeared over the years, lost to encroaching vegetation from a combination of lack of use and no trail maintenance.

 MILESTONES

▶1	0.0	Start at trailhead
▶2	1.75	Little Baldy summit

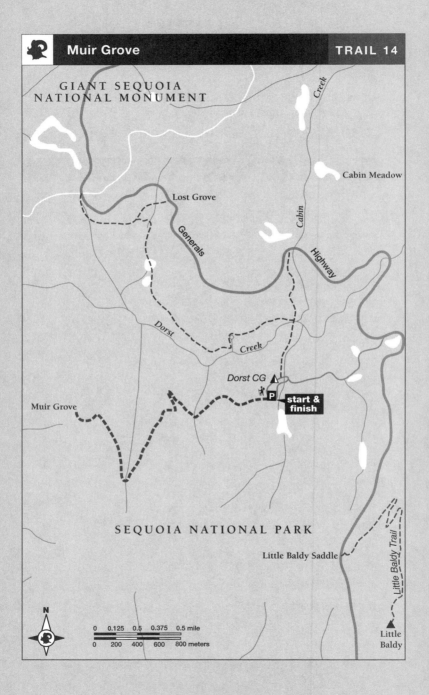

Muir Grove — TRAIL 14

GIANT SEQUOIA NATIONAL MONUMENT

Creek

Cabin Meadow

Lost Grove

Generals

Cabin

Highway

Dorst

Creek

Dorst CG

Muir Grove

P start & finish

SEQUOIA NATIONAL PARK

Little Baldy Saddle

Little Baldy Trail

N

0   0.125   0.5   0.375   0.5 mile
0   200   400   600   800 meters

Little Baldy

Muir Grove

Off the beaten path and tucked away from hordes of tourists who frequent the more popular groves of giant sequoias, Muir Grove is a rare gem. The nearly 1-mile drive from the Generals Highway when combined with the 2-mile hike to the grove seems enough of a deterrent to keep the crowds at bay and allow hikers the opportunity to stand among the Big Trees with a strong possibility for peace and serenity. John Muir should be pleased to have his name attached to this quiet grove of stately trees.

Best Time

Since the trailhead is located nearly a mile inside Dorst Campground, the best time to hike this trail is between Memorial Day and Labor Day weekends, when the campground is open. The dogwood flowers are usually showy in late spring, followed by the wildflower bloom in early summer. If you don't mind adding an extra 1.8 miles round-trip to walk the road, autumn can be a fine time for this hike, when the campground is closed, virtually no one is on the trail, and the dogwood leaves are ablaze with color—a fine complement to the red bark of the sequoias.

Finding the Trail

From Visalia, follow Highway 198 to Three Rivers and proceed east into Sequoia National Park, where the road becomes Generals Highway. Drive on Generals Highway to the entrance into Dorst Campground (fee, flush toilets, running water,

TRAIL USE
Dayhike

LENGTH
4.2 miles, 2 hours

VERTICAL FEET
+535/-515/±2100

DIFFICULTY
– 1 2 **3** 4 5 +

TRAIL TYPE
Out & Back

FEATURES
Fall Colors
Giant Sequoias
Great Views
Secluded

FACILITIES
Campground
Restrooms

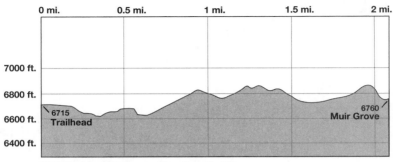

TRAIL 14 Muir Grove Elevation Profile

bear boxes, and phone), 8 miles northwest of the Lodgepole turnoff (17.3 miles southeast of the Y-junction with Highway 180). Proceed on the main access road through the campground 0.9 mile to the signed trailhead and then continue to the parking lot near the campground amphitheater. Wuksachi Village, a short distance north of Lodgepole, offers upscale lodging and dining. Stony Creek Village and Montecito Lake Resort are slightly less expensive lodging options.

Off the beaten path and tucked away from hordes of tourists who frequent the more popular groves of giant sequoias, Muir Grove is a rare gem.

Trail Description

▶1 Begin the hike by walking back down the road from the parking lot to the start of the trail near a small metal sign marked MUIR GROVE TRAIL. Immediately cross a log bridge over a delightful tributary of Dorst Creek and then make a mild descent through mixed forest to a junction. ▶2

Turn sharply left at the junction and traverse around a hillside well above the main channel of the creek to the crossing of another tributary. A moderate ascent follows, aided by a couple of switchbacks, leading to the crest of a ridge and an exposed granite hump, where the trees part enough to allow a fine view of Chimney Rock, Big Baldy, and the densely forested drainages of Stony and

Dorst creeks. The confluence of these two streams, within rugged and virtually inaccessible terrain, is the birthplace of the North Fork Kaweah River. Careful observation from this vantage across the canyon will reveal the crowns of giant sequoias extending above the lesser conifers.

Great Views

Leaving the granite hump behind, you proceed in and out of a mixed forest of firs, pines, and cedars on a mildly undulating traverse to the crossing of a flower-lined tributary of Dorst Creek. From there, the mildly ascending trail leads to the top of a ridge, passing azaleas and dogwoods along the way, which provide striking colors in fall. Just beyond, you reach the first of the sequoias, a pair of burned remnants and a massive giant just off the trail. A short distance farther is perhaps the highlight of **Muir Grove**, ▶3 a circle of a dozen or more giant sequoias arranged in a nearly symmetrical pattern. Standing among this ring of Goliaths stirs a feeling of reverential awe fitting for such a grand cathedral. Short, faint paths lead away from this magical spot to additional sequoias scattered about, but the old trail that once continued on to Skagway Grove, Hidden Spring, and North Fork Kaweah River is overgrown and very hard, if not impossible, to follow.

Fall Colors

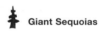

Giant Sequoias

𝝠	MILESTONES	
▶1	0.0	Start at trailhead
▶2	0.2	Turn left at junction
▶3	2.1	Muir Grove

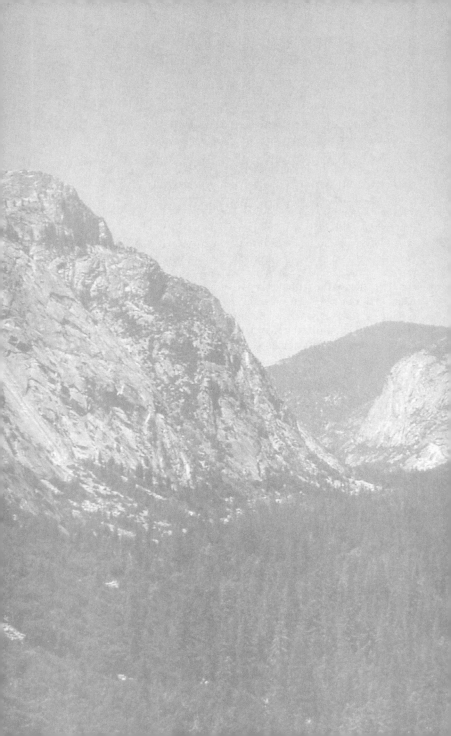

West Kings Canyon

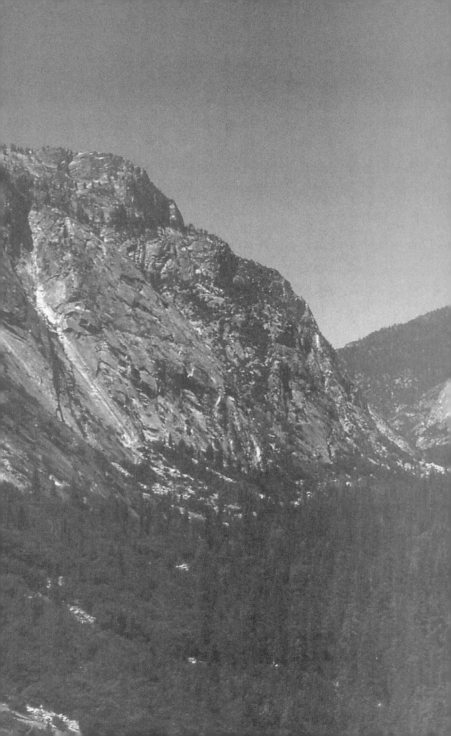

West Kings Canyon

The west side of the Sierra Nevada rises slowly but steadily from the broad plain of the San Joaquin Valley toward the federally protected lands of Sequoia National Park. Traveling east, the verdant and productive agricultural lands of the San Joaquin Valley gradually transition into the oak-dotted grasslands and chaparral of the foothills zone, followed by a sea of green from the dense timber of the mid-elevation forests. Fortunately, only a few roads penetrate this area of towering conifers and isolated groves of giant sequoias, and auto-bound tourists are completely blocked from access to the granite cirques, alpine meadows, and jagged peaks associated with the High Sierra. Steadily rising, roadless wilderness continues through the red fir and lodgepole pine forests into the subalpine and alpine zones before climaxing at the Sierra Crest, along the eastern border of the park.

Visitors entering Kings Canyon from the west experience a wide range of topography, flora, and fauna. The west side of the park has two major hubs of activity, **Grant Grove,** home to some of the world's largest sequoias, and **Kings Canyon**, one of the deepest gorges in North America. The first three trails in this section are outside of these two areas, with principal access provided by Generals Highway. Trail 15 is a short climb to superb views from one of the park's western domes. The largest collective grove of giant sequoias, **Redwood Grove**, provides the site for Trail 16. Trail 17 is within Jennie Lakes Wilderness, offering a short but stiff climb to the summit of **Mitchell Peak**, another fine vista point. Trails 18–20 wander through Grant Grove to waterfalls, scenic vistas, and giant sequoias. **Converse Basin** is the setting for Trail 21, a short hike to one of the largest giant sequoias in existence, a survivor of logging that almost completely decimated the basin of the Big Trees. The remaining trails, 22–27, all originate from the deep gorge of **Kings Canyon**, where hikers are treated to panoramic vistas, waterfalls, South Fork Kings River, and the majesty of one of the deepest canyons in North America, a less famous counterpart to Yosemite Valley.

Overleaf and opposite: *Kings Canyon View, Bubbs Creek Trail*

Permits

Permits are not required for dayhikes. Backpackers must obtain a wilderness permit for all overnight visits in the park. From trips between the Thursday before Memorial Day and the last Sunday in September, permits are based on a quota system and cost $15 per party. Off-season permits are free and available by self-registration. Up to 75 percent of the quota can be reserved between March 1 and September 10 (applications submitted outside of these dates will not be processed). Complete and submit a downloadable application (www.nps.gov/seki) with the $15 nonrefundable fee (Visa, MasterCard, check, or money order) by mail or fax. Applications must be received before 14 days prior to the first day of a trip. Walk-in permits may be obtained after 1 PM the day before entry from the Grant Grove Visitors Center or the Roads End Wilderness Cabin. Unclaimed reservations become available for walk-in permits after 9 AM on the day of entry.

Maps

For West Kings Canyon, the USGS 7.5-minute (1:24,000 scale) topographic maps are listed below.

> Trails 15–16: *General Grant Grove*
> Trail 17: *Muir Grove, Mt. Silliman*
> Trails 18–20: *General Grant Grove*
> Trail 21: *Hume*
> Trail 22: *Cedar Grove*
> Trail 23: *The Sphinx*
> Trail 24: *Cedar Grove*
> Trails 25–26: *The Sphinx*
> Trail 27: *Cedar Grove*

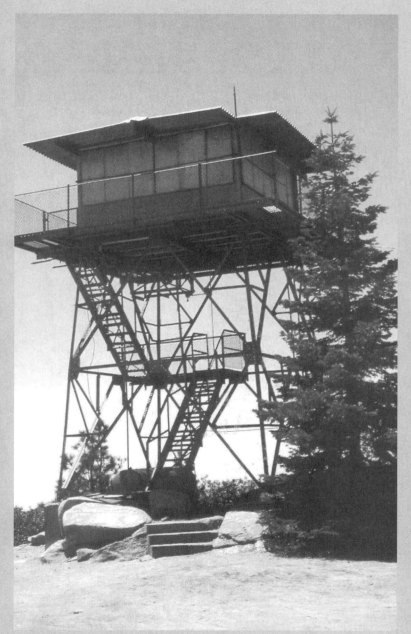

Park Ridge Lookout *(Trail 20)*

West Kings Canyon

15	Big Baldy	**22**	Lookout Peak
16	Redwood Mountain Grove	**23**	Roaring River Falls
17	Mitchell Peak	**24**	Zumwalt Meadow Nature Trail
18	Sunset Loop Trail	**25**	Kanawyer Loop Trail
19	General Grant Tree Trail	**26**	Mist Falls
20	Panoramic Point and Park Ridge Lookout	**27**	Hotel and Lewis Creeks Loop
21	Boole Tree		

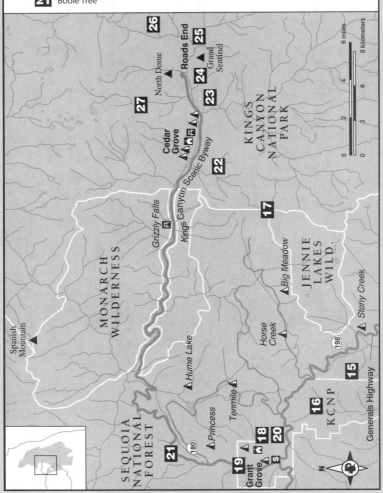

West Kings Canyon

TRAIL	Difficulty	Length	Type	USES & ACCESS	TERRAIN	FLORA & FAUNA	OTHER
15	3	4.4	Out & Back	Dayhiking, Running	Summit		Great Views
16	3	7.25, 6.6	Loop	Dayhiking, Backpacking, Running		Fall Colors, Wildflowers, Giant Sequoias	Great Views, Camping, Secluded
17	4	6.0	Out & Back	Dayhiking, Running	Mountain, Summit	Wildflowers	Great Views, Secluded, Steep
18	3	6.4	Loop	Dayhiking, Running	River or Stream, Waterfall	Wildflowers, Giant Sequoias	Great Views
19	1	0.5	Loop	Dayhiking, Child Friendly, Handicapped Access		Giant Sequoias	
20	2	5.6	Loop	Dayhiking, Running			Great Views
21	2	4.5	Loop	Dayhiking		Giant Sequoias	Great Views
22	4	10.0	Out & Back	Dayhiking, Running	Mountain, Summit	Wildflowers	Great Views, Steep
23	1	0.5	Out & Back	Dayhiking	Waterfall		
24	1	1.5	Loop	Dayhiking, Child Friendly	River or Stream		Great Views
25	2	4.7	Loop	Dayhiking, Running, Horses, Child Friendly	River or Stream		Great Views, Fishing
26	3	7.8	Out & Back	Dayhiking, Running, Horses	Canyon, River or Stream, Waterfall		Fishing
27	4	6.4	Out & Back	Dayhiking, Running, Horses	Canyon, River or Stream	Wildflowers	Great Views

USES & ACCESS
- Dayhiking
- Backpacking
- Running
- Horses
- Dogs Allowed
- Child Friendly
- Handicapped Access

TYPE
- Loop
- Out & Back

DIFFICULTY
- 1 2 3 4 5 +
less   more

TERRAIN
- Canyon
- Mountain
- Summit
- Lake
- River or Stream
- Waterfall

FLORA & FAUNA
- Fall Colors
- Wildflowers
- Giant Sequoias

FEATURES
- Great Views
- Camping
- Swimming
- Secluded
- Steep
- Historic Interest
- Fishing

West Kings Canyon

Panoramic Point
and Park Ridge Lookout......... 153

Gently graded segments of single-track trail and fire road lead hikers from one fantastic vista at Panoramic Point to another one at Park Ridge Lookout. Still operational, Park Ridge is one of the few remaining fire lookouts from a former network that once spanned the length and breadth of the Sierra.

TRAIL 20

Dayhike, Run
5.6 miles, Loop
Difficulty: 3

Boole Tree 157

The decimation of hundreds of giant sequoias in Converse Basin is one of the great travesties of a bygone era. Amid this devastation stands the spared Boole Tree, eighth largest giant sequoia in the world. A fine loop trail leads to this massive survivor, with good views of the Kings River gorge on the return.

TRAIL 21

Dayhike
4.5 miles, Loop
Difficulty: 2

Lookout Peak 161

Follow the Don Cecil Trail on a stiff climb from Cedar Grove to one of the park's best views of Kings Canyon from the summit of Lookout Peak. The 4000-foot elevation gain may be taxing, but the amazing vista is a more than adequate reward for all the hard work.

TRAIL 22

Dayhike, Run
10.0 miles, Out & Back
Difficulty: 4

Roaring River Falls 165

Before Roaring River empties into South Fork Kings River near Cedar Grove, the waters spill down the south wall of Kings Canyon in a pair of scenic falls. A very short stroll leads to a viewpoint of the lower falls, a magnificent sight, especially in late spring when the river is swollen with snowmelt from the high mountains above.

TRAIL 23

Dayhike
0.5 mile, Out & Back
Difficulty: 1

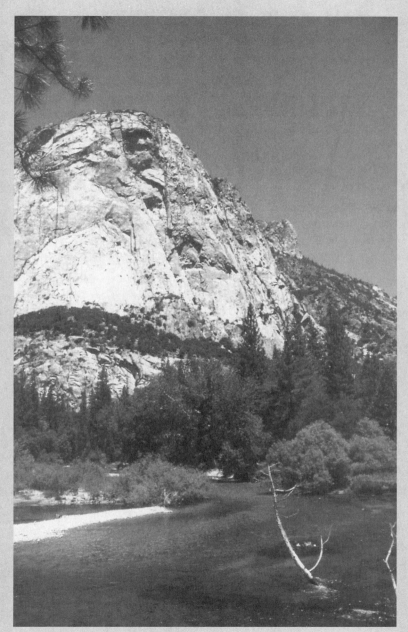

North Dome, *Kings Canyon (Trail 24)*

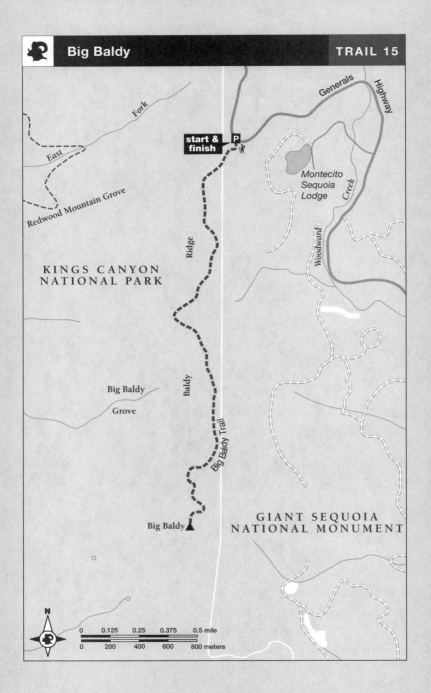

Big Baldy

TRAIL 15

start &
finish

P

Generals

Highway

East

Fork

Montecito
Sequoia
Lodge

Creek

Redwood Mountain Grove

Woodward

Ridge

KINGS CANYON
NATIONAL PARK

Baldy

Big Baldy

Grove

Big Baldy Trail

Big Baldy ▲

GIANT SEQUOIA
NATIONAL MONUMENT

N

0   0.125   0.25   0.375   0.5 mile

0   200   400   600   800 meters

Big Baldy

Several granite domes rise above the forested terrain on the west side of Kings Canyon and Sequoia national parks, offering inspirational views to those who can gain their summits. At 8209 feet, Big Baldy is one such dome, offering hikers a 360-degree view east toward the Sierra and west across the San Joaquin Valley as the reward for a mere 2.2-mile trip to the summit. Bring along plenty of water, as none is available at the trailhead or along the trail.

Best Time

Snow melts from the Big Baldy Trail by the beginning of June in years of average snowfall. As with most vista points on the west side of the parks, the view across the San Joaquin Valley is best following a rare cleansing rainstorm.

Finding the Trail

From Fresno, drive Highway 180 to the Y-junction with the Generals Highway, turn right and follow Generals Highway 6.3 miles to the start of the Big Baldy Trail (16.9 miles northwest of Lodgepole). Park your vehicle along the shoulder of the highway as space allows. Giant Sequoia National Monument has a number of campgrounds not far from the trailhead, including Stony Creek (fee, flush toilets, running water, and bear boxes) accessed from Generals Highway, and Horse Camp (vault toilets and no fee), Buck Rock (vault toilets and no fee), and Big Meadow (vault toilets, phone, and no fee) accessed from Big Meadow Road. Privately run

TRAIL USE
Dayhike, Run

LENGTH
4.4 miles, 2 hours

VERTICAL FEET
+975/-450, ±2850

DIFFICULTY
- 1 2 **3** 4 5 +

TRAIL TYPE
Out & Back

FEATURES
Summit
Great Views

FACILITIES
None

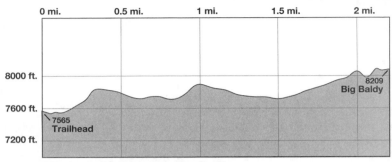

| 0 mi. | 0.5 mi. | 1 mi. | 1.5 mi. | 2 mi. |

8000 ft.

8209
Big Baldy

7600 ft.

7565
Trailhead

7200 ft.

TRAIL 15 Big Baldy Elevation Profile

Montecito Lake Resort is a year-round lodge about 1 mile from the trailhead just off Generals Highway. Stony Creek Village (guest rooms, market, restaurant, showers, and gasoline) is about 4 miles farther southbound on Generals Highway.

Trail Description

▶1 From the vicinity of a wood trail sign on the west side of the highway, follow single-track trail through a sparse fir forest, soon crossing the boundary into Kings Canyon National Park and following near the crest of an undulating, south-trending ridge. From the top of a granite outcrop, about a half mile from the trailhead, the trees part enough to allow a fine view down into neighboring **Redwood Canyon**.

On a rare clear day, the view extends all the way west to the coastal hills.

Continue along the ridge for the next 1.5 miles, passing in and out of light mixed forest, with the sporadic openings offering a tantalizing foretaste of the view waiting ahead at the top of Big Baldy. Nearing the summit, you pass below a television tower and a concrete block building before a final, winding ascent over rocks leads to the top of the exposed granite dome. ▶2

 Summit

The view from the apex of **Big Baldy** is grand indeed, with the serrated summits of peaks belonging to the Kings-Kaweah and Great Western divides

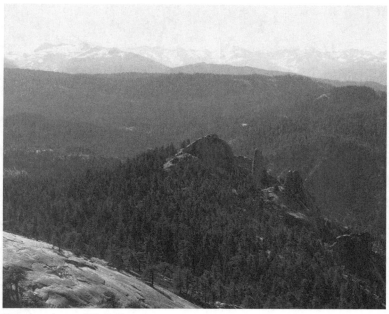

View *from the top of Big Baldy*

beyond Little Baldy to the east. Westward, across Redwood Canyon and Redwood Mountain, lie the foothills and the usually smoggy air above the San Joaquin Valley. On a rare clear day, the view extends all the way west to the coastal hills.

 Great Views

🚶	MILESTONES	
▶1	0.0	Start at trailhead
▶2	2.2	Big Baldy

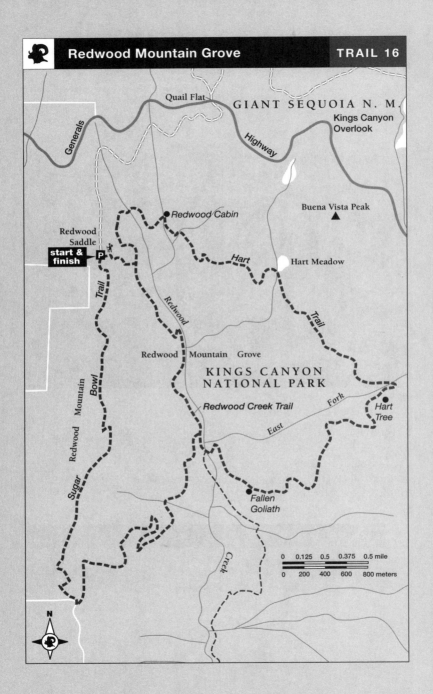

Quail Flat

GIANT SEQUOIA N. M.

Kings Canyon
Overlook

Generals

Highway

Redwood Cabin

Buena Vista Peak

Redwood
Saddle

start &
finish   P

Hart   Hart Meadow

Trail

Redwood

Trail

Redwood   Mountain   Grove

KINGS CANYON
NATIONAL PARK

Redwood   Mountain

Bowl

Redwood Creek Trail

East   Fork

Hart
Tree

Sugar

Fallen
Goliath

Creek

0	0.125	0.5	0.375	0.5 mile
0	200	400	600	800 meters

N

Redwood Mountain Grove

The largest intact grove of giant sequoias in the world would be, you would think, a very popular destination. However, the trails within the Redwood Mountain Grove are lightly used, perhaps due to the absence of a paved road, or lack of a motorized tram similar to the one that transports tourists through the Mariposa Grove in Yosemite. Thankfully, this magnificent grove of giant sequoias can be fully appreciated sans crowds while walking beneath the towering monarchs in relative tranquility.

The Redwood Grove has a network of trails that can be combined into a couple of fine loop trips. In addition to the magnificent redwoods found along either circuit, the Hart Trail Loop visits a number of enchanting brooks lined with ferns and wildflowers. Most of the trip passes through cool forest, but occasionally the trees part enough to reveal pleasant views of the surrounding peaks, such as at Hart Meadow, where the verdant clearing is stunningly backdropped by the west face of Buena Vista Peak. The slightly shorter Sugar Bowl Loop has some unique features as well, including an interesting work in progress—a hillside carpeted with Christmas-tree-size sequoias on the site of an old burn. A pleasant stroll down lushly lined Redwood Creek is well complemented by a traverse of Redwood Mountain, from where you have excellent views of Big Baldy and Buena Vista Peak, two stately granite domes. Backpackers can travel farther downstream along Redwood Creek to fine streamside campsites (two-night limit, no fires).

TRAIL USE
Dayhike, Backpack, Run
LENGTH
7.25 miles, 4 hours
6.6 miles, 3½ hours
VERTICAL FEET
+2065/-2065/±4130
+2130/-2130/±4260
DIFFICULTY
− 1 2 **3** 4 5 +
TRAIL TYPE
Loop

FEATURES
Fall Colors
Wildflowers
Giant Sequoias
Great Views
Camping
Secluded

FACILITIES
Restrooms

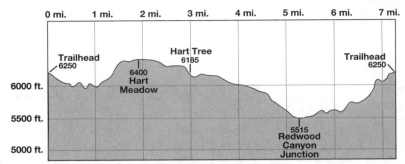

TRAIL 16 Redwood Mountain: Hart Trail Loop Elevation Profile

Best Times

By the end of April or beginning of May, the trails of Redwood Grove shed their covering of winter snow. Somewhat off the beaten path, the trails are host to the highest number of visitors between Fourth of July and Labor Day weekend. Springtime offers the added bonus of blooming dogwoods, while fall offers leaves ablaze with autumn color.

Finding the Trail

From Fresno, follow Highway 180 to the Y-junction with the Generals Highway, turn right and follow Generals Highway 3.4 miles to Quail Flat. Directly opposite Tenmile Road, turn south and follow a narrow dirt road with turnouts for 1.7 miles to a junction. Bear left at the junction signed for Redwood Mountain Grove, and after 0.1 mile come to the entrance to the large parking area at Redwood Saddle. Tenmile and Landslide (fee and vault toilets) are U.S. Forest Service campgrounds located nearby along Tenmile Road.

Trail Description

HART TRAIL LOOP: ▶1 From the trailhead, take the left-hand trail signed HART TREE, REDWOOD CANYON TRAIL and head north, descending into a mixed forest of firs, pines, and giant sequoias, while following the course of an old roadbed to a junction in a small ravine. ▶2 Bear left and proceed under cool and shady forest on soft dirt tread past lush ground cover, winding down to an easy boulder-hop of a wildflower- and fern-lined tributary of Redwood Creek. From the creek a mild climb leads to the next delightful, flower-lined branch, where you can see Redwood Cabin above the far bank.

 Fall Colors

 Wildflowers

The climb continues away from the cabin for another 0.2 mile to yet another stream crossing. Leave the stream and most of the redwoods behind, as the trail climbs more moderately. Through infrequent gaps in the forest, you catch fleeting glimpses of Redwood Mountain to the west before reaching a granite outcrop with an unobstructed view of the mountain and Big Baldy to the southeast. A mild climb from the outcrop leads to the fringe of Hart Meadow, ▶3 a sloping, verdant glade picturesquely backdropped by the west face of Buena Vista Peak. After stepping across the twin channels of Buena Vista Creek, you bid farewell to this pastoral scene.

 Fire Ecology

NOTE

Over the last few decades, biologists have learned a great deal about the relationship between fire and the giant sequoia through experimental burns performed in research areas within the Redwood Mountain Grove. For instance, the thick bark of sequoias protects them from the ravages of a forest fire while other conifer species are burned, thereby creating space on the forest floor for new sequoia saplings. The tiny sequoia cone also releases its seeds when heated by a fire.

In addition to the magnificent redwoods found along either circuit, the Hart Trail Loop visits a number of enchanting brooks lined with ferns and wildflowers.

A general descent leads away from the meadow and back into the mighty presence of the Big Trees, reaching the Fallen Tunnel Tree, where the trail passes directly through the hollowed core of this downed giant sequoia. The mostly gentle descent continues through the cool forest, eventually drawing alongside a trickling seasonal stream followed by lushly lined East Fork Redwood Creek, spilling serenely over moss-covered rocks and swirling gently through diminutive pools—a quite pleasant forest scene. A brief climb from the East Fork brings you to a junction with a short spur to the Hart Tree, ▶4 one of the 20 largest giant sequoias in the world. Black scars 20 to 30 feet up the trunk provide evidence that this immense redwood has withstood some significant fires in the past.

Gently descending tread leads away from the Hart Tree spur past a thin ribbon of water from a seasonal stream cascading down a rock cleft into a pool lined with lush foliage and wildflowers. Proceed through a mixed forest of incense cedars, white firs, and a smattering of sequoias, interrupted briefly by a sunny clearing filled with drier vegetation, on the way to a junction with a spur to a huge downed sequoia known as the **Fallen Goliath**. ▶5

Another half mile leads to a crossing of the main branch of Redwood Creek, a crossing that could prove a little difficult in early season. Just over the creek you reach a junction with the **Redwood Creek Trail**, ▶6 where backpackers could head downstream a short distance to campsites farther down the canyon.

 Camping

Turn right and head upstream along the Redwood Canyon Trail on a mild climb through a mixed forest that includes towering sequoias, soon passing a junction with the **Sugar Bowl Trail** on your left. ▶7 The lushly lined trail continues upstream for another ¾-mile before forsaking the creek to climb across a hillside on the way to a junction ▶8 at the

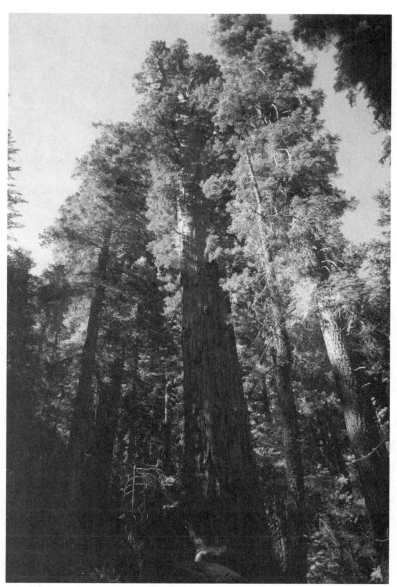

Hart Tree, *Redwood Canyon*

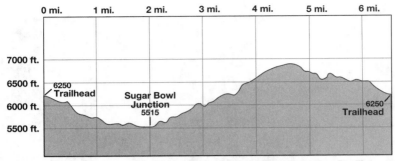

TRAIL 16 Redwood Mountain: Sugar Bowl Loop Elevation Profile

close of the loop section. From there, retrace your steps back to the trailhead at **Redwood Saddle**. ▶9

SUGAR BOWL LOOP: From the trailhead, take the left-hand trail signed HART TREE, REDWOOD CANYON TRAIL and head north, descending into a mixed forest of firs, pines, and giant sequoias, while following the course of an old roadbed to a junction in a small ravine. ▶2 Bear right at the junction and follow the **Redwood Creek Trail** initially on a gentle descent that soon becomes moderate. A mile or so from the junction, you reach the west bank of enchanting Redwood Creek and proceed downstream through lush vegetation past a number of stately giant sequoias. The path stays reasonably close to the creek for a while, veers away briefly, and then follows the stream to a junction with the **Sugar Bowl Trail**. ▶3

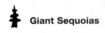

Giant Sequoias

Turn right and head southwest from the junction on a moderate climb up a hillside. Beyond a pair of short-legged switchbacks, you continue the climb across a slope covered with myriad young sequoias and dotted by a few widely scattered old giants. Over the tops of the young trees, the granite dome of Big Baldy puts in an appearance. Cross a seasonal stream, where the increase in moisture has given rise to more mature trees that provide a pocket of welcome shade. Beyond the stream the moderate ascent continues across open slopes via a set of switchbacks

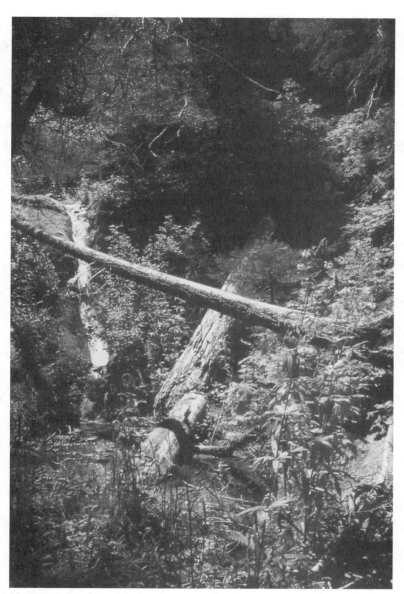

Rivulet *in Redwood Mountain Grove*

climbing across a hillside covered with drought-tolerant shrubs, such as manzanita and huckleberry oak. As you climb, views continue to improve of Big Baldy, Buena Vista Peak, and the surrounding terrain. The moderate climb abates where the trail gains the crest of Redwood Mountain's lengthy ridge.

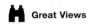 **Great Views**

Now the trail turns north and follows the ridge into the cover of a mixed forest, where giant sequoias once again tower over their lower counterparts. As you proceed amid these majestic monarchs on soft tread, you may eventually notice the end of the Big Trees near the east end of the ridge, further evidence that sequoias require specialized conditions for their growth and survival. Most likely the soil on this side of the ridge doesn't receive a suitable amount of moisture for the sequoias to flourish. Climb mildly to the high point of the journey, weaving in and out of forest cover along the way, where good views from the clearings span across Redwood Canyon to the granite domes of **Buena Vista Peak** and **Big Baldy**. A gradual descent leads away from the high point through mixed forest to close the loop at the parking area. ►4 From there, retrace your steps to the trailhead at **Redwood Saddle**.

MILESTONES

Hart Trail Loop

▶1   0.0   Head left at trailhead
▶2   0.3   Bear left at junction
▶3   1.9   Hart Meadow
▶4   3.0   Hart Tree
▶5   4.75   Fallen Goliath
▶6   5.25   Turn right at Redwood Canyon junction
▶7   5.3   Straight at Sugar Bowl junction
▶8   6.9   Turn right at junction
▶9   7.25   End at trailhead

Sugar Bowl Loop

▶1   0.0   Head left at trailhead
▶2   0.3   Bear right at junction
▶3   2.0   Turn right at Sugar Bowl junction
▶4   6.6   End at trailhead

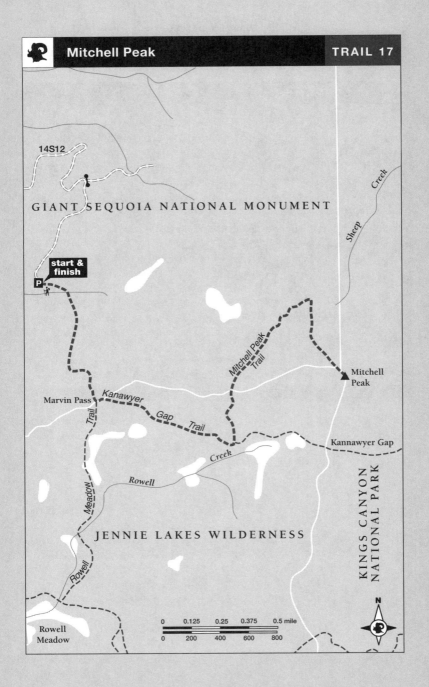

14S12

GIANT SEQUOIA NATIONAL MONUMENT

Sheep Creek

start & finish

P

Mitchell Peak Trail

Mitchell Peak

Marvin Pass

Kanawyer Gap Trail

Kannawyer Gap

Trail

Creek

Meadow

Rowell

KINGS CANYON NATIONAL PARK

JENNIE LAKES WILDERNESS

Rowell

| 0 | 0.125 | 0.25 | 0.375 | 0.5 mile |

| 0 | 200 | 400 | 600 | 800 |

N

Rowell Meadow

Mitchell Peak

Mitchell Peak is a seldom-visited mountain situated on the border between Jennie Lakes Wilderness and Kings Canyon National Park, and the summit affords one of the best viewpoints accessible by maintained trail on the western side of the parks. You can enjoy the ascent and the summit views of the Sierra Crest, Great Western Divide, Kaweah Peaks, and the deep gorge of Kings Canyon with a reasonable expectation of solitude.

Best Times

Hikers can scale snow-free trails to the summit of Mitchell Peak usually from the middle of June until the first storm of the season, generally at the end of October or in early November.

Finding the Trail

From Fresno, follow Highway 180 to the Y-junction with the Generals Highway, turn right and follow Generals Highway 9.7 miles to a left-hand turn onto Big Meadows Road. Proceed east for 10.3 miles past Horse Camp Campground (vault toilets and no fee) and Big Meadow Campground (vault toilets, phone, and no fee) to the signed turnoff for the Marvin Pass Trailhead on the right and drive another 3.1 miles on dirt road to the trailhead (staying on the main road at all intersections).

Trail Description

▶1 Head past the trailhead register and proceed uphill on single-track tread through a mixed forest of white firs, lodgepole pines, and western white

TRAIL USE
Dayhike, Run
LENGTH
6.0 miles, 3–4 hours
VERTICAL FEET
+2000/±4000
DIFFICULTY
– 1 2 3 **4** 5 +
TRAIL TYPE
Out & Back

FEATURES
Mountain
Summit
Wildflowers
Great Views
Secluded
Steep

FACILITIES
None

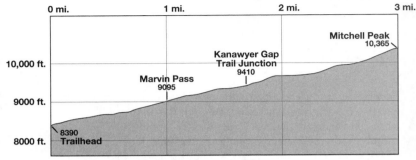

TRAIL 17 Mitchell Peak Elevation Profile

pines and an assortment of shrubs, including manzanita, chinquapin, and currant. A moderately steep
climb leads to the top of a ridge, where the ascent
eases a bit and then continues to a junction ►2 with
a lateral to **Sequoia High Sierra Camp**, a hike-in
resort one-third mile to the east. Proceed ahead
from the junction and immediately cross a small
fern- and flower-lined rivulet. Pass above a pocket
of lush foliage dotted with an array of wildflowers
that includes shooting star, corn lily, buttercup, and
monkeyflower. Away from these lush surroundings, the steady ascent continues via switchbacks to
the signed wilderness boundary and a junction at
Marvin Pass. ►3

> Leaving the last of
> the trees behind,
> you weave your
> way southeast
> among boulders to a
> commanding view on
> top of Mitchell Peak.

Head southeast on the **Kanawyer Gap Trail**
across the south side of a ridge through scattered to
light forest, as well as shrubs and boulders, where
lupine and paintbrush add splashes of color in early
season. A mellow traverse leads to a junction in a
field of chinquapin. ►4

Turn left (north) and ascend a mostly open
slope back up and across the ridgecrest, and then
veer northeast to follow an ascending traverse across
the northwest side of Mitchell Peak through a light,
mixed forest of western white pines, red firs, and
lodgepole pines. Eventually the grade increases on
a winding climb toward the block summit of the

peak. Leaving the last of the trees behind, you weave your way southeast among boulders to a commanding view on top of **Mitchell Peak**. ▶5

Perhaps the most impressive sight from the summit is the foreground terrain plummeting steeply northeast into the deep cleft of **Kings Canyon**, backdropped majestically by the rising profile of the Monarch Divide. A vast array of Sierra summits can be seen as well, including the Palisades and Mt. Goddard along the northeastern horizon, a multiplicity of summits along the **Great Western Divide**, and the multicolored **Kaweah Peaks** to the southeast. Fragments of the old fire lookout are scattered about the summit, a silent reminder that rangers once had the privilege of enjoying this remarkable view daily.

 Great Views

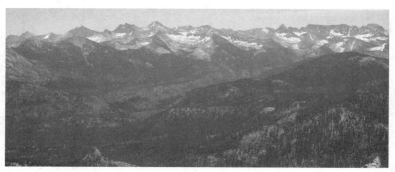

View *from Mitchell Peak*

🚶	**MILESTONES**	
▶1	0.0	Start at parking area
▶2	0.4	Straight at Sequoia High Sierra Camp Junction
▶3	1.0	Turn left at Marvin Pass junction
▶4	1.7	Turn left at junction
▶5	3.0	Mitchell Peak

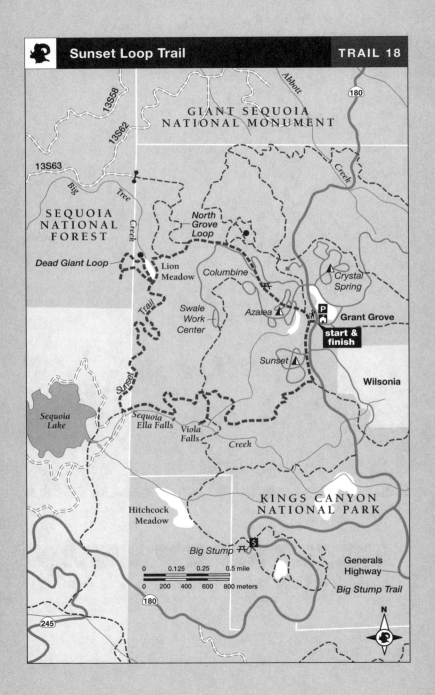

Sunset Loop Trail

Waterfalls, vistas, and big trees are the prime attractions for this trip through a section of Grant Grove, an area with far fewer visitors than around General Grant Tree. Ella and Viola falls put on a showy display in late spring and early summer, when Sequoia Creek is running high from snowmelt. Added treats include an overlook offering a grand view of Sequoia Lake and, of course, the opportunity to see some notable giant sequoias.

Best Time

Hikers will usually find the trails in Grant Grove to be free of snow from late May to mid-October.

Finding the Trail

Follow Highway 180 east from Fresno into Kings Canyon National Park and continue to Grant Grove Village. Park your vehicle in the visitors center parking lot. Grant Grove has three campgrounds, Azalea, Crystal Springs, and Sunset (fee, flush toilets, and bear boxes). John Muir and Grant Grove lodges offer hotel rooms and cabins, and the village has a restaurant, showers, general store, and gift shop, as well as a visitors center.

Trail Description

▶1 To locate the start of the Sunset and Azalea trails, follow the crosswalk directly opposite the visitors center across Highway 180 to the west side of the road and a trail sign. A very short path leads

TRAIL USE
Dayhike, Run
LENGTH
6.4 miles, 3 hours
VERTICAL FEET
+1885/-1885/±3770
DIFFICULTY
– 1 2 **3** 4 5 +
TRAIL TYPE
Loop

FEATURES
Streams
Waterfalls
Wildflowers
Giant Sequoias
Great Views

FACILITIES
Lodging
Store
Cafe
Visitors Center
Post Office
Restrooms
Water
Picnic Area
Campgrounds
Stables

141

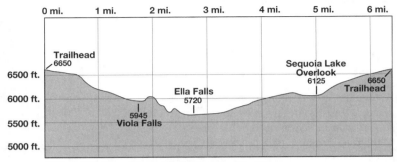

TRAIL 18 Sunset Loop Trail Elevation Profile

downhill from there to a marked junction, ►2 where you turn left to follow a trail that parallels the highway toward Sunset Campground. Soon cross the campground access road and proceed to a T-junction between the Azalea and Sunset trails. ►3

Turn right and follow the **Sunset Trail** over a low hill and then make a short descent on indistinct tread to the bottom of a swale. After a very brief climb away from the swale, break out into a small clearing, where the trail is lined with manzanita. From the clearing the route of the trail becomes more obvious again, as you begin a steady descent that lasts until the park boundary near Sequoia Lake. Weave down the hillside over slabs and around boulders through a light, mixed forest to a bridge over a tributary of Sequoia Creek and continue to a signed, four-way junction with an old road from the Swale Work Center. ►4

Turn left (south) at the junction and follow the old road on a mild descent through moderate forest for 0.2 mile to where the road bends east. A small sign marked VIOLA FALLS directs foot traffic straight ahead onto single-track trail that soon leads alongside **Sequoia Creek**. The narrow and somewhat faint path ends at the base of a hill, from where you can work your way to an overlook directly above **Viola Falls**. ►5 Don't expect the scenic drama of a

Waterfall

Yosemite-type waterfall, as Viola Falls is more like a series of cataracts pouring swiftly down a narrow channel into the swirling pools of basins that have been scoured out of solid rock. Early season wildflowers add a lovely touch of color to the stream banks.

 Wildflowers

Retrace your steps back to the four-way junction ▶6 and turn left toward **Ella Falls**. A steady descent through light to moderate forest leads to a series of switchbacks that take you across a seasonal stream, over a seep, and down to Ella Falls. ▶7 While Viola Falls may seem a bit tame, Ella presents the sights and sounds one expects from a significant waterfall. In spring and early summer, Sequoia Creek plunges raucously down a sh eer face into a whirling pool before resuming a cacophonous journey toward Sequoia Lake.

 Waterfall

Proceed a quarter mile beyond Ella Falls to a junction ▶8 between the boundary of Kings Canyon National Park and the private property of the YMCA camps around Sequoia Lake. The YMCA has granted permission to pass over their land to hikers who wish to continue ahead a short distance to an overview of the lake. Those who choose to do so should remain on the trail and out of the camps.

Following a sign marked GRANT TREE, angle away from the trail to Sequoia Lake and follow the continuation of the Sunset Trail on a moderately steep climb to an old road ▶9 that used to be the main access into the park via Sequoia Lake. Once at the

Sequoia Lake

HISTORY

Although at first glance the body of water before you appears natural, Sequoia Lake was created in the late 1800s as a millpond to provide water for a flume that carried lumber to a mill in Sanger in the San Joaquin Valley below. Today the lake is home to a number of summer camps.

road, turn right and proceed on broken asphalt on a steady, winding ascent that leads through the partial shade of a mixed forest. Pass by a couple of roads on the left coming from the vicinity of the lake and continue the climb to the top of a hill and a junction with the **Dead Giant Loop Trail** on the left, ▶10 4.75 miles from the trailhead.

Turn left at the junction and follow the lower part of the Dead Giant Loop across a lightly forested hillside above verdant Lion Meadow. Continue a short distance past the far edge of the meadow to the Dead Giant, a very large sequoia that met an untimely demise at the hands of axe-wielding loggers. Careful inspection of the trunk reveals axe marks encircling the trunk that basically sheared off the cambium layer, permanently interrupting the flow of nutrients up the tree. Without such life-giving sustenance, the tree eventually succumbed, providing a visual memorial to modern-day visitors of an age-old truth: Nature's greatest enemy is man himself. Leaving the Dead Giant behind, climb a hillside to the crest of an open ridge and then follow this spine southwest to an unmarked junction. ▶11 Continue straight ahead a short distance to where the ridge begins to fall away, soon arriving at **Sequoia Lake Overlook**.

After fully enjoying the view, backtrack the short distance to the junction ▶12 and, following a sign marked simply TRAIL, proceed eastbound on the return leg of the loop back to the junction with the **Sunset Trail**. ▶13

From the Dead Giant Loop junction, resume the climb along the old roadbed, passing around the edge of Lion Meadow. After 0.25 mile you pass the first junction ▶14 of the North Grove Trail and then the second junction ▶15 0.25 mile farther. A short distance from the second junction, you reach the edge of a large parking lot for the popular **General Grant Tree area**. Stroll across the lot to the far side

While Viola Falls may seem a bit tame, Ella presents the sights and sounds one expects from a significant waterfall.

and the resumption of trail near a restroom building and a grove of sequoias known as the **Happy Family**, passing the General Grant trailhead along the way.

Giant Sequoias

Walk along a split-rail fence just to the left of Big Tree Creek, a delightful rivulet lined with

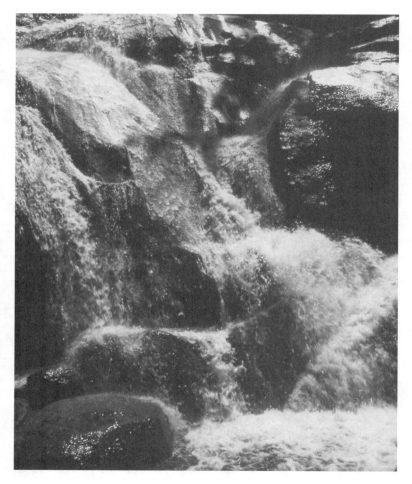

Ella Falls

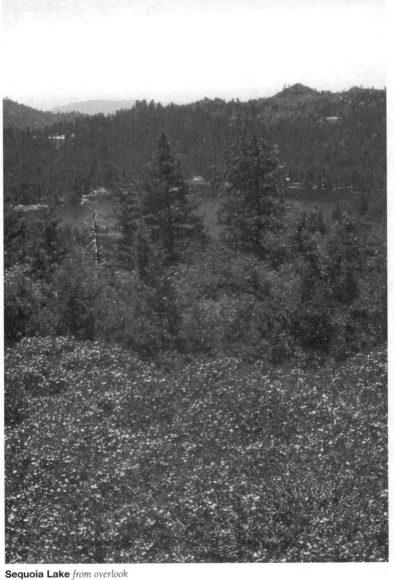

Sequoia Lake *from overlook*

verdant plants. Cross the tiny stream on a wood plank bridge and pass by the **Michigan Tree**, a huge, toppled-over giant sequoia that lies in broken sections beside the trail. The fence ends just beyond the tree, but you continue up the trail to a crossing of the Giant Tree road. A short climb through light forest away from the road leads past Columbine Picnic Area and into Azalea Campground. Pass through the campground, negotiating a number of access road crossings, walk across a plank bridge, and then ascend the hillside to the junction across from the visitors center at the close of your loop. ▶16 From there, retrace your steps the short distance to the parking lot. ▶17

🚶	**MILESTONES**	
▶1	0.0	Start at Grant Grove Visitors Center
▶2	0.01	Left at junction
▶3	0.3	Right at Azalea-Sunset junction
▶4	1.5	Left at junction
▶5	1.75	Viola Falls
▶6	2.0	Left at junction
▶7	2.75	Ella Falls
▶8	3.0	Right at junction
▶9	3.03	Right at old road
▶10	4.75	Left at Dead Giant junction
▶11	5.0	Straight ahead at Sequoia Lake Overlook junction
▶12	5.05	Veer left at junction
▶13	5.4	Left at Sunset Trail junction
▶14	5.65	Straight at first North Grove Trail junction
▶15	5.9	Straight at second North Grove Trail junction
▶16	6.39	Left at junction
▶17	6.4	End at Grant Grove Visitors Center

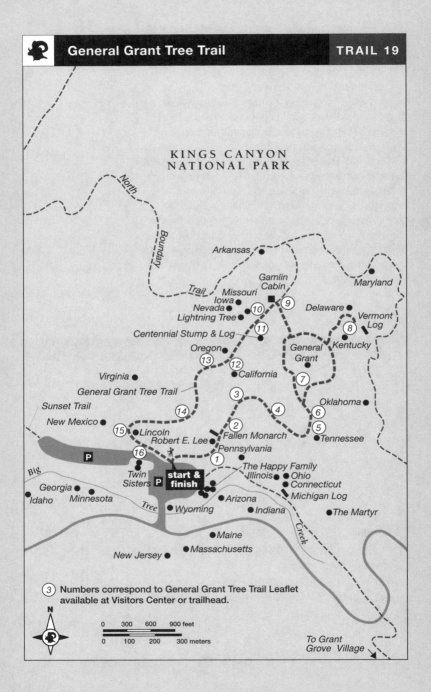

KINGS CANYON
NATIONAL PARK

North

Boundary

Trail

Arkansas

Gamlin Cabin

Maryland

Missouri
Iowa
Nevada ⑩ ⑨ Delaware
Lightning Tree Vermont Log
Centennial Stump & Log ⑪ ⑧
Oregon General Kentucky
⑬ ⑫ Grant
California ⑦
Virginia
General Grant Tree Trail Oklahoma
③
Sunset Trail ④ ⑥
New Mexico ⑤
⑮ Lincoln ⑭ Tennessee
Robert E. Lee ② Oklahoma
Big ⑯ Fallen Monarch
Pennsylvania
Twin Sisters ① The Happy Family
Georgia start & Illinois Ohio
Idaho Minnesota finish Connecticut
Tree Wyoming Arizona Michigan Log
Indiana The Martyr
Maine
New Jersey Massachusetts

③ Numbers correspond to General Grant Tree Trail Leaflet
available at Visitors Center or trailhead.

N

| 0 | 300 | 600 | 900 feet |
| 0 | 100 | 200 | 300 meters |

To Grant
Grove Village

General Grant Tree Trail

With a height of 268 feet and a base diameter of more than 40 feet (as measured in 2002), the General Grant Tree has the distinction of being the third largest living tree in the world. Additional prestige is attached to the Grant Grove area as being the oldest parcel of land in Kings Canyon National Park, set aside as General Grant National Park in 1890 by the same congressional bill that established Yosemite National Park and greatly enlarged Sequoia National Park. Such notoriety has resulted in making Grant Grove one of the area's most popular tourist attractions and the easy half-mile loop around the namesake tree one of the area's most popular trails. Be sure to pick up a leaflet at the visitors center or the trailhead.

Best Time

While the trail is generally free of snow from mid-May to mid-October, weekends between the Fourth of July and Labor Day see big crowds. Even weekdays can be very busy during that period, with hordes of tourists craning their necks to see the namesake tree. During peak season an early morning or early evening visit may alleviate the congestion somewhat.

Finding the Trail

Follow Highway 180 east from Fresno and, just north of the Grant Grove Visitors center, turn west at the well-signed junction with the road to the General Grant Tree. Follow the access road 0.7

TRAIL USE
Dayhike, Child Friendly, Handicapped Access
LENGTH
0.5 mile, ½ hour
VERTICAL FEET
+100/-100/±200
DIFFICULTY
− 1 **2** 3 4 5 +
TRAIL TYPE
Loop

FEATURES
Giant Sequoias

FACILITIES
Lodging
Store
Cafe
Visitors Center
Post Office
Restrooms
Water
Picnic Area
Campgrounds
Stables

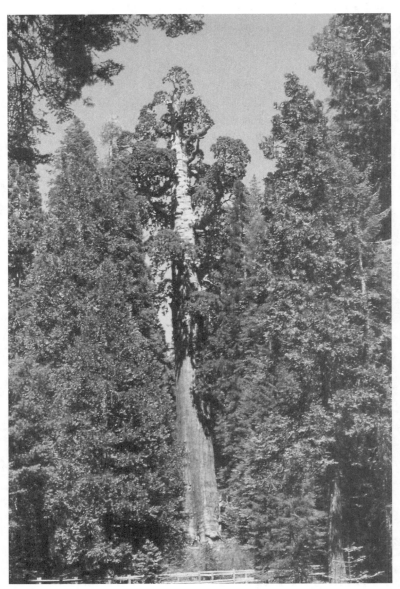

General Grant Tree

mile to the large parking lot. Grant Grove has three campgrounds, Azalea, Crystal Springs, and Sunset (fee, flush toilets, and bear boxes). John Muir and Grant Grove lodges offer hotel rooms and cabins, and the village has a restaurant, showers, general store, and gift shop.

Trail Description

▶1 Head in a counterclockwise direction on the paved loop trail, weaving your way up to the area's centerpiece attraction, the **General Grant Tree**. ▶2 A short climb from this immense monarch takes you past the **Gamlin Cabin**, followed by a mild descent beside more giant sequoias back to the trailhead. Trail extensions north of the grove are far less traveled, providing options for further wanderings.

⋀	MILESTONES		
▶1	0.0	Begin at trailhead	
▶2	0.2	Walk around General Grant Tree	

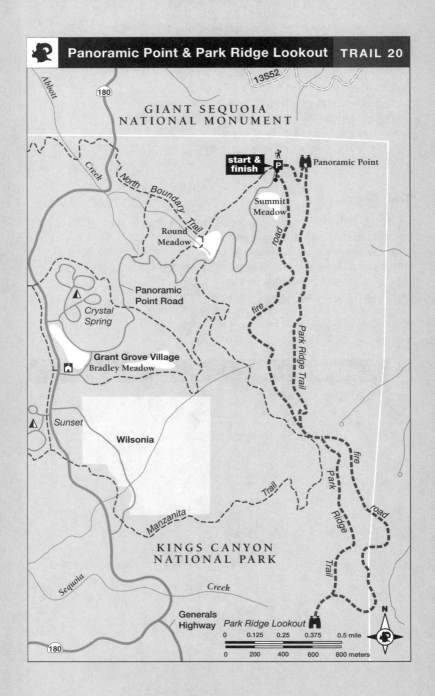

GIANT SEQUOIA
NATIONAL MONUMENT

13S52

180

Abbott

Creek

North Boundary Trail

Round Meadow

start & finish

P

Panoramic Point

Summit Meadow

fire road

Panoramic Point Road

Crystal Spring

Grant Grove Village
Bradley Meadow

Sunset

Wilsonia

Park Ridge Trail

Manzanita Trail

Park Ridge Trail

fire road

KINGS CANYON
NATIONAL PARK

Sequoia

Creek

Generals Highway

Park Ridge Lookout

180

0   0.125   0.25   0.375   0.5 mile

0   200   400   600   800 meters

N

Panoramic Point and Park Ridge Lookout

This fine trip begins with a short walk to the view-packed tourist destination of Panoramic Point, where visitors are treated to outstanding views of the Great Western Divide, Sierra Crest, and Monarch Divide. From there, the pleasant loop combines a hiking trail and a fire road to access one of the few remaining operational fire lookouts in the Sierra, where hikers will have far fewer elbows to rub while admiring vistas of the Great Western Divide and San Joaquin Valley. Alternating between mixed forest and shrub-covered clearings, the route along Park Ridge is fairly gently graded.

Best Time

The view from Panoramic Point is extraordinary at any time of the year, although you may need cross-country skis or snowshoes in winter. Hikers will find snow-free trails to the lookout from late May through October.

Finding the Trail

From Fresno, follow Highway 180 east into Kings Canyon National Park and, just north of the Grant Grove Visitors Center, turn east at the well-signed junction with Panoramic Point Road. Proceed on paved road for 2.3 miles to the trailhead. Restrooms and a picnic area are nearby. Grant Grove has three campgrounds, Azalea, Crystal Springs, and Sunset (fee, flush toilets, and bear boxes). John Muir and Grant Grove lodges offer hotel rooms and cabins, and the village has a restaurant, showers, general store, and gift shop.

TRAIL USE
Dayhike, Run

LENGTH
5.6 miles, 2½–3 hours

VERTICAL FEET
+1430/-1430/±2860

DIFFICULTY
– 1 **2** 3 4 5 +

TRAIL TYPE
Loop

FEATURES
Great Views

FACILITIES
Lodging
Store
Cafe
Visitors Center
Post Office
Restrooms
Water
Picnic Area
Campgrounds
Stables

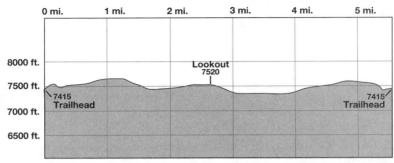

TRAIL 20   Panoramic Point and Park Ridge Lookout Elevation Profile

Trail Description

▶1 Follow paved trail bordered by a split rail fence for about 300 yards to Panoramic Point, ▶2 where a magnificent view unfolds. Metal signs help identify some of the numerous peaks of the Monarch Divide, Great Western Divide, and Sierra Crest seen from this spectacular vista point.

Leaving the vast majority of sightseers behind, you continue up the trail away from Panoramic Point, following a winding climb that weaves in and out of scattered to light forest, with an understory of manzanita and azalea. Scarred trunks on many of the conifers provide evidence of a recent fire. Where the forest parts, views northeast of the Monarch Divide alternate with views southeast of the Great Western Divide, and views west toward San Joaquin Valley. Reach the crest of a knoll past the 1-mile mark and then begin a moderate descent to a junction where the trail merges with a fire road at 1.6 miles. ▶3

Walk along the fire road for about 50 yards to a signed junction with the resumption of single-track trail. ▶4 The trail follows a mildly undulating course for another mile before merging with the fire road again. ▶5 Follow the road for approximately 250 yards to the vicinity of the fire lookout tower,

Great Views

The view from the lookout—from the San Joaquin Valley to the Great Western Divide and points in between—is quite rewarding.

▶6 where transformers, power poles, communication towers, weather monitoring equipment, and a concrete block building litter the edge of the ridge. Despite the human-made features, the view from the lookout—from the San Joaquin Valley to the Great Western Divide and points in between—is quite rewarding.

Great Views

After fully enjoying the view, retrace your steps 250 yards to the trail junction ▶7 and veer right to continue along the Fire Road. Proceed on the gently graded road through a light, mixed forest, wrapping around a hillside above Log Corral Meadow to the junction with the single-track trail that heads south toward the lookout. ▶8 Continue on the road another 50 yards to the next junction ▶9 of single-track trail and, remaining on the road, you make a general ascent for about 0.8 mile across open slopes dotted with fire-scarred trees and covered with shrubs. A final half-mile descent leads past a small meadow to a closed gate. From there, follow a short stretch of paved road back to the parking lot. ▶10

🚶 MILESTONES

▶1	0.0	Start at trailhead
▶2	0.1	Panoramic Point
▶3	1.6	Straight at fire road
▶4	1.63	Straight at junction
▶5	2.7	Straight at fire road
▶6	2.75	Lookout
▶7	2.8	Veer right at junction
▶8	4.05	Straight at junction
▶9	4.1	Straight at junction
▶10	5.6	Return to trailhead

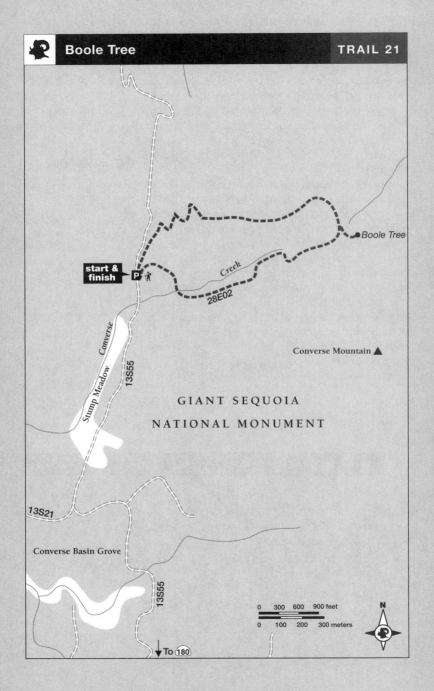

Boole Tree

start & finish

Creek

28E02

Converse Mountain ▲

GIANT SEQUOIA

NATIONAL MONUMENT

Stump Meadow

Converse

13S55

13S21

Converse Basin Grove

13S55

| 0 | 300 | 600 | 900 feet |

| 0 | 100 | 200 | 300 meters |

N

To 180

Boole Tree

Hikers can travel a short distance on this trail into Converse Basin to marvel at the eighth largest giant sequoia in the world. Along the way, eight other conifer species may be observed, including lodgepole, western white, Jeffrey, and sugar pines, as well as red and white firs and incense cedars. In addition to the trees, the section of the loop beyond the Boole Tree provides excellent views down into the canyon of South Fork Kings River.

Best Time

The Boole Tree makes an excellent short hike anytime between late May and November.

Finding the Trail

Follow Highway 180 east from Fresno to the Big Stump Entrance into Kings Canyon National Park and continue past Grant Grove Village to Forest Road 13S55, about 4.25 miles north of Grant Grove. Drive 0.25 mile to a triple junction and proceed straight ahead (remaining on FS 13S55) through Stump Meadow to the trailhead parking area, 2.5 miles from Highway 180. Princess Campground (fee, vault toilets, and running water) is about 3 miles eastbound on Highway 180 from the junction with 13S55.

Trail Description

►1 Pass through a wood gate and walk uphill through a thick canopy of mixed forest. Continue on a moderate climb on switchbacks and up log steps, followed by a short descent to a T-junction.

TRAIL USE
Dayhike

LENGTH
4.5 miles, 2–2½ hours

VERTICAL FEET
+750/-750/±1500

DIFFICULTY
– 1 **2** 3 4 5 +

TRAIL TYPE
Loop

FEATURES
Giant Sequoias
Great Views

FACILITIES
Restroom
Picnic Area

Boole Tree

Sometimes size has advantages, and such was the case with the Boole Tree. While hundreds of giant sequoias met the ax in Converse Basin, this lone survivor received a stay of execution due to its great size. Considered at one time to be the third largest sequoia in existence, the Boole Tree was spared the fate of its less fortunate neighbors. Although this impressive monarch has the largest base circumference of any sequoia (113 feet), a height of 269 feet and volume of 42,472 cubic feet ultimately ranked the tree as the eighth largest in the world. Ironically, the tree was named for Frank Boole, the Converse Basin mill superintendent who oversaw the demise of the rest of the giant sequoias in the area.

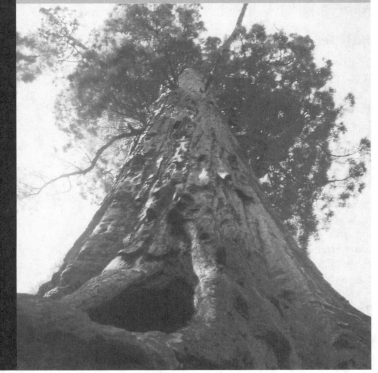

Boole Tree

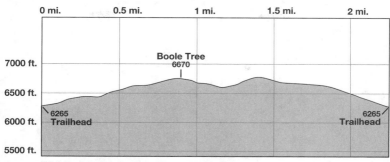

TRAIL 21 Boole Tree Elevation Profile

A very short descent from the junction leads to the massive **Boole Tree**. ▶2

After fully admiring the huge monarch, return to the junction and ascend a hillside to a viewpoint overlooking the deep gorge of Kings River. You might notice a significant change in foliage to more drought-tolerant plants like manzanita, mountain misery, and scattered Jeffrey pine on the hilltop. Heading west, follow a ridge downhill to a series of switchbacks, with more fine views of the Kings River country along the way. The descent continues southwest back to the parking area. ▶3

While hundreds of giant sequoias met the ax in Converse Basin, this lone survivor received a stay of execution due to its great size.

🚶	**MILESTONES**	
▶1	0.0	Start at trailhead
▶2	0.9	Boole Tree
▶3	4.5	End at trailhead

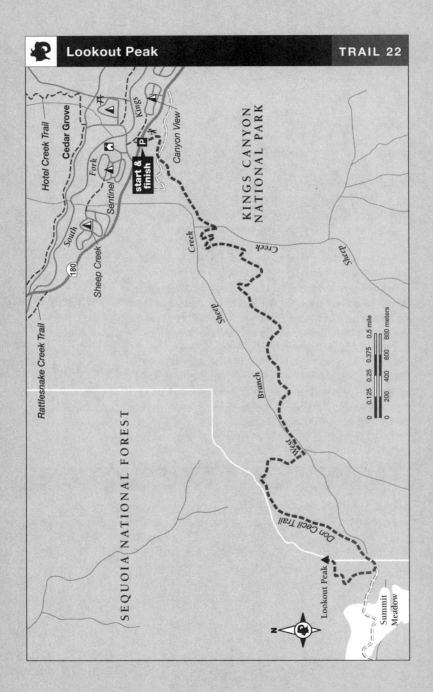

Lookout Peak — TRAIL 22

KINGS CANYON NATIONAL PARK

SEQUOIA NATIONAL FOREST

Cedar Grove

Hotel Creek Trail

Rattlesnake Creek Trail

Kings

Canyon View

start & finish

South Fork

Sentinel

Sheep Creek

180

Creek

Creek

Sheep

Sheep

West Branch

Don Cecil Trail

Lookout Peak

Summit Meadow

N

0   0.125   0.25   0.375   0.5 mile
0   200   400   600   800 meters

Lookout Peak

This trip follows the Don Cecil Trail to the top of Lookout Peak, from which hikers have a bird's-eye view of the deep cleft of Kings Canyon and an impressive vista of the peaks and ridges in the backcountry of Kings Canyon National Park. While a few tourists may hike the first part of the trail to the cool grotto of Sheep Creek, the remaining 4 miles of trail sees little use—a definite bonus for solitude seekers. The steady, 4000-foot climb seems more than enough to deter the average park visitor. Although stiff, the ascent can be done in a few hours by hikers in reasonable condition. Be sure to shoot for an early start, however, as temperatures at these relatively low elevations can become hot during the heat of the day.

Best Time

The route to the 8485-foot summit is usually free of snow from June to mid-October. Wildflowers along Sheep Creek are usually at their peak sometime in early summer.

Finding the Trail

From Fresno, follow Highway 180 east into Kings Canyon National Park and continue past Grant Grove into Kings Canyon. Park your vehicle along the shoulder of the highway near the trailhead, 0.15 mile east of the turnoff into Cedar Grove. The Park Service has four campgrounds in the Cedar Grove area: Sentinel, Sheep Creek, Canyon View, and Moraine (all of which have fees, flush toilets, running water, and bear boxes). Cedar Grove has a motel, showers, general store, restaurant, and laundry facilities.

TRAIL USE
Dayhike, Run

LENGTH
10.0 miles, 5 hours

VERTICAL FEET
+4000/-225/±8450

DIFFICULTY
– 1 2 3 **4** 5 +

TRAIL TYPE
Out & Back

FEATURES
Mountain
Summit
Wildflowers
Great Views
Steep

FACILITIES
Lodging
Store
Visitors Center
Snack Bar
Restrooms
Showers
Laundromat
Water
Picnic Area
Campgrounds
Stables

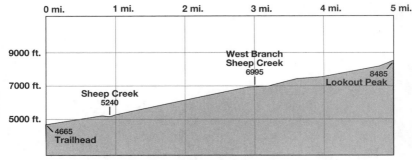

TRAIL 22   Lookout Peak Elevation Profile

Trail Description

▶1 The trail begins by climbing the south wall of the canyon on a moderately steep grade through a light, mixed forest of black oaks, incense cedars, ponderosa pines, and white firs. Careful perusal of the trunks reveals black scars, indicating that this area has seen its share of forest fires. Soon the trail bends west to cross an access road for the Cedar Grove heliport and then resumes the stiff ascent before shortly dropping to **Sheep Creek** at 0.9 mile, ▶2 where the cool and refreshing waters cascade picturesquely down a series of rock slabs. As Sheep Creek is the domestic water source for Cedar Grove, do not contaminate the water in any way. Fortunately for solitude seekers, most sightseers go no farther than the bridge over the creek.

Beyond the creek, a series of switchbacks lead through scattered forest, with periodic breaks that allow fine views of Kings Canyon below, the Monarch Divide to the north, and the Sierra Crest to the east—precursors of the much more excellent view waiting at the top of Lookout Peak. The forest thickens a tad on the approach to the west branch of Sheep Creek, which is lined with a verdant assortment of wildflowers, ferns, and small plants. After a short stroll alongside this pleasant stream, you cross the creek on a flat-topped log. ▶3

> Nearly 4000 feet straight below is the South Fork Kings River, tumbling through the rugged and deep gorge of Kings Canyon.

After following the north bank for a while, the trail veers away from the creek and then climbs across the east slope of Lookout Peak through more drought-tolerant vegetation. A protracted climb leads to a saddle at the **signed boundary of Kings Canyon National Park and Sequoia National Forest**. ▶4

 Steep

Beyond the boundary, the condition of the trail deteriorates to a faint path that leads up to the crest of the peak's west ridge and then follows the ridge to the summit. In the absence of well-defined tread, small ducks may help guide you up the ridge, but the route is quite obvious. The path becomes more distinct again, as the trail dips shortly, winds across a shrub-covered slope, and then zigzags toward the summit. Nearing the top, pick your way around large slabs and over boulders to emerge triumphantly on top of **Lookout Peak**. ▶5

 Summit

Although a large microwave telephone reflector anchored to the top of the peak may detract from the sense of wildness, the view is nonetheless dramatic. Nearly 4000 feet straight below is the South Fork Kings River, tumbling through the rugged and deep gorge of Kings Canyon. Across the canyon to the north, the Monarch Divide cuts a jagged profile across the azure Sierra sky. Looking east, the peaks of the Sierra Crest span the horizon. If you're fortunate enough to be here on a rare, clear day following a cleansing summer rain, even the view across the San Joaquin Valley can be impressive.

 Great Views

🚶	**MILESTONES**	
▶1	0.0	Start at trailhead
▶2	0.9	Sheep Creek
▶3	3.0	West Branch Sheep Creek
▶4	4.3	Saddle at park boundary
▶5	5.0	Lookout Peak

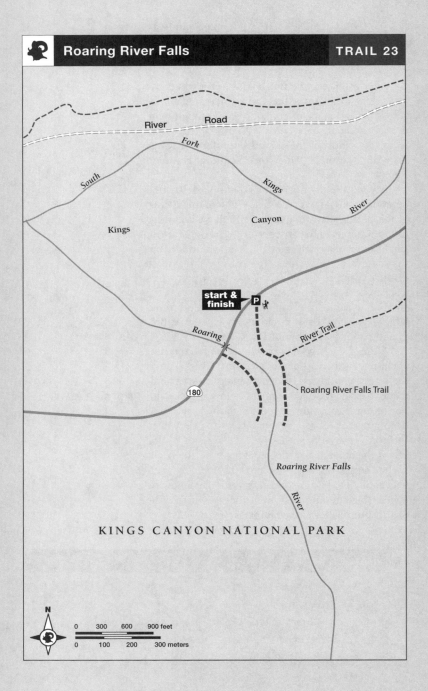

Roaring River Falls

TRAIL 23

River Road

South Fork

Kings

Canyon

Kings River

start & finish

P

Roaring

River Trail

180

Roaring River Falls Trail

Roaring River Falls

River

KINGS CANYON NATIONAL PARK

N

| 0 | 300 | 600 | 900 feet |
| 0 | 100 | 200 | 300 meters |

Roaring River Falls

While the short trip to a view of Roaring River Falls is not much of a hike by most standards, the falls are impressive and should be seen at least once by anyone visiting Kings Canyon.

Best Times

While the highway into Cedar Grove is open from late April to mid-November, Roaring River Falls can be best appreciated in late spring and early summer, when snowmelt in the higher elevations swells Roaring River into a wild torrent and the falls into a turbulent, raging, two-tiered cascade. However, the falls are still reasonably scenic later in the season, as Roaring River always seems to have a dependable supply of water.

Finding the Trail

From Fresno, follow Highway 180 east into Kings Canyon National Park and continue past Grant Grove into Kings Canyon. Drive 2.8 miles past the Cedar Grove turnoff to the signed parking area on the right. The Park Service has four campgrounds in the Cedar Grove area: Sentinel, Sheep Creek, Canyon View, and Moraine (all of which have fees, flush toilets, running water, and bear boxes). Cedar Grove has a motel, showers, general store, restaurant, and laundry facilities.

TRAIL USE
Dayhike
LENGTH
0.5 mile, ¼ hour
VERTICAL FEET
+100/-100/±200
DIFFICULTY
– **1** 2 3 4 5 +
TRAIL TYPE
Out & Back

FEATURES
Waterfall

FACILITIES
Lodging
Store
Visitors Center
Post Office
Restrooms
Water
Picnic Area
Campgrounds
Stables

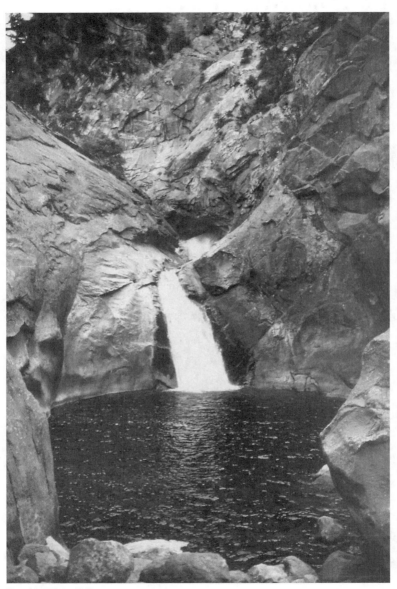

Roaring River Falls

Trail Description

▶1 Follow a paved path away from the parking area on the east side of Roaring River through mixed forest and foliage typical of Kings Canyon. A short, mild climb leads to a junction with the River Trail on the left, where you continue straight ahead a short distance to **a viewpoint of the falls**. ▶2

 Waterfall

An alternate route heads west from the parking area and across the highway bridge to the start of dirt tread on the west side of Roaring River. The path heads above the west bank to a series of rock steps that lead down to a fenced viewpoint.

🚶	MILESTONES	
▶1	0.0	Start at trailhead
▶2	0.25	Roaring River Falls viewpoint

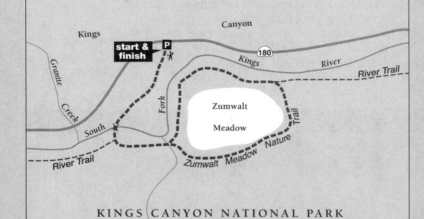

Kings

Canyon

start & finish

P

180

Kings

River

River Trail

Granite

Creek

Fork

South

Zumwalt

Meadow

Trail

River Trail

Zumwalt Meadow Nature

KINGS CANYON NATIONAL PARK

N

0   300   600   900 yards

0   100   200   300 meters

Zumwalt Meadow Nature Trail

The easy 1.5-mile loop around Zumwalt Meadow provides a leisurely way to get acquainted with the ecology of Kings Canyon. An inexpensive pamphlet filled with interesting tidbits about the natural history of the immediate area is a fine complement to the journey around the meadow. Along with surveys of the verdant, grass- and flower-filled meadow, the short path offers plenty of additional scenery, from glimpses of the scenic South Fork Kings River to impressive views of the glistening granite spires and cliffs on the canyon walls, including Grand Sentinel and North Dome.

Best Time

The road into Kings Canyon is usually open from late May to mid-November, with the majority of tourists visiting the area between Memorial Day and Labor Day weekends. South Fork Kings River is a raging torrent in late spring, when the meadow grass is green and wildflowers add splashes of color. Summer temperatures can be hot; an afternoon dip in the reduced river flow offers a refreshing alternative for beating the heat. Autumn, when many of the tourists are gone and the weather is pleasant, can be a fine time for a visit as well.

Finding the Trail

From Fresno, follow Highway 180 east into Kings Canyon National Park and continue past Grant Grove into Kings Canyon. Continue up-canyon to

TRAIL USE
Dayhike, Child Friendly
LENGTH
1.5 miles, 1 hour
VERTICAL FEET
+100/-100/±200
DIFFICULTY
– **1** 2 3 4 5 +
TRAIL TYPE
Loop

FEATURES
Stream
Great Views

FACILITIES
Lodging
Store
Visitors Center
Post Office
Restrooms
Water
Picnic Area
Campgrounds
Stables

the Zumwalt Meadow parking lot, 4.25 miles east of the turnoff to Cedar Grove. The Park Service has four campgrounds in the Cedar Grove area: Sentinel, Sheep Creek, Canyon View, and Moraine (all of which have fees, flush toilets, running water, and bear boxes). Cedar Grove has a motel, showers, general store, restaurant, and laundry facilities.

Trail Description

▶1 Your first stop along the Zumwalt Meadow Nature Trail should be at the trailhead signboard, where, for a nominal fee, you can purchase a pamphlet with a map and detailed information corresponding to the 18 numbered posts placed along the self-guiding trail. Once you're armed with a pamphlet, follow a wide path to a suspension bridge spanning South Fork Kings River. Along the way and on the bridge, you have fine views of verdant Zumwalt Meadow, the river, and Grand Sentinel rising sharply above the canyon floor. Immediately beyond the bridge is a junction with the **River Trail**. ▶2

Turn left (east) and proceed upstream on the River Trail through cool forest, soon arriving at the westernmost junction with the **Zumwalt Meadow Nature Trail**. ▶3 Proceed straight ahead at the junction, leaving the forest canopy behind to follow a

Along the way and on the bridge, you have fine views of verdant Zumwalt Meadow, the river, and Grand Sentinel.

HISTORY

Daniel K. Zumwalt

Daniel K. Zumwalt was a land agent and attorney for the Southern Pacific Railroad who, along with his employee, Jesse Agnew, acquired 120 acres of land near Cedar Grove. Zumwalt was a strong advocate for preserving the natural heritage of the area, influencing the decision to set aside land for General Grant (subsequently incorporated into the much larger Kings Canyon National Park) and Sequoia national parks in 1890. Nowadays this meadow bears the name of one of the park's most influential advocates.

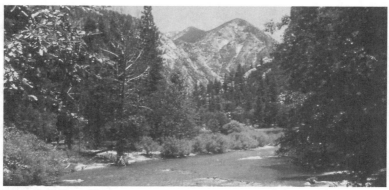

South Fork Kings River

brief climb across an exposed talus field above the
meadow. From this slightly higher vantage, you
have fine views across the meadow and the river
to the far canyon wall. Soon reach the easternmost
junction of the nature trail. ►4

Great Views

Turn left at the junction, leaving the River Trail
to skirt the fringe of the grassy meadow on the way
toward the riverbank. Then follow the meandering
river downstream, aided by a section of boardwalk,
to the close of the loop at the westernmost junction
of the nature trail. ►5 From there, retrace your steps
to the junction near the bridge. ►6 Turn right at the
junction, cross the bridge, and then retrace your
steps back to the parking lot. ►7

MILESTONES

►1	0.0	Start at trailhead
►2	0.25	Left at junction
►3	0.35	Straight at junction
►4	0.65	Left at junction
►5	1.1	Right at junction
►6	1.25	Right at junction
►7	1.5	End at trailhead

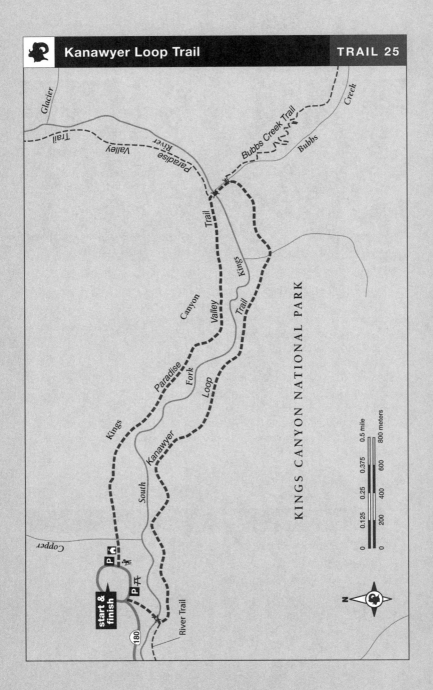

KINGS CANYON NATIONAL PARK

start & finish

Kanawyer Loop Trail

Roads End is a very popular trailhead for the army of recreationists bound for trips into the heart of the southern Sierra. Chances are you will share the first half of this loop trip with plenty of backpackers, dayhikers, and equestrians headed for popular destinations accessed by the Paradise Valley and Bubbs Creek trails. However, on the second half of the journey the troops drop off considerably, allowing the notion of quiet solitude in the upper end of Kings Canyon to be a real possibility. The loop is an easy stroll across the nearly level valley floor, making this a trip well suited for hikers at any level of skill and fitness. Be prepared for hot afternoon temperatures in summer, but relief via a refreshing dip in the chilly waters of South Fork Kings River is never too far away.

Best Time

The road into Kings Canyon is usually open from late May to mid-November, with the majority of tourists visiting the area between Memorial Day and Labor Day weekends. South Fork Kings River is a raging torrent in late spring, when the meadow grass is green and wildflowers add splashes of color. Summer temperatures can be hot; an afternoon dip in the reduced river flow offers a refreshing alternative for beating the heat. Autumn, when many of the tourists are gone and the weather is pleasant, can be a fine time for a visit as well.

TRAIL USE
Dayhike, Run, Horse, Child Friendly

LENGTH
4.7 miles, 2½ hours

VERTICAL FEET
+275/-275/±550

DIFFICULTY
– 1 **2** 3 4 5 +

TRAIL TYPE
Loop

FEATURES
Stream
Great Views
Fishing

FACILITIES
Lodging
Store
Visitors Center
Post Office
Restrooms
Water
Picnic Area
Campgrounds
Stables

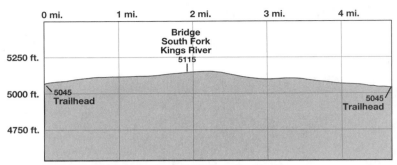

TRAIL 25   Kanawyer Loop Trail Elevation Profile

Finding the Trail

The loop is an easy stroll across the nearly level valley floor, making this a trip well suited for hikers at any level of skill and fitness.

From Fresno, follow Highway 180 east into Kings Canyon National Park and continue past Grant Grove into Kings Canyon. Continue up-canyon to the day-use parking area at Roads End, 5.0 miles east of the turnoff to Cedar Grove. The Park Service has four campgrounds in the Cedar Grove area: Sentinel, Sheep Creek, Canyon View, and Moraine (all of which have fees, flush toilets, running water, and bear boxes). Cedar Grove has a motel, showers, general store, restaurant, and laundry facilities.

Trail Description

From the parking area, walk to the **well-signed trailhead ►1** at the east end of the paved turnaround at Roads End, near the rustic cabin that serves as the wilderness permit office. Follow a wide, sandy, gently ascending path that parallels the river through a mixed forest of incense cedars, ponderosa pines, black oaks, sugar pines, and white firs to a bridge across Copper Creek. Continue up-canyon into thinning forest cover, with occasional views of the impressive granite walls of Kings Canyon, which are often compared favorably to the more famous walls of Yosemite Valley. Soon you enter a shady forest of ponderosa pines, sugar pines, white firs, and alders on the way to a Y-junction with the **Paradise Valley Trail**. ▶2

Turn right (south) at the junction and immediately cross a bridge over the river, just downstream from its confluence with Bubbs Creek. Soon you reach another junction, ▶3 this one between the **Bubbs Creek Trail** headed southeast and the Kanawyer Trail headed southwest.

Turn right and follow the **Kanawyer Trail**, where you may notice evidence of a recent fire. Cross Avalanche Creek on a pair of logs and follow gently graded trail through dense forest. Past a small meadow, the trail draws closer to the south bank of the river, where anglers can easily drop a line. As you continue downstream, the forest parts just enough on occasion to allow grand views of the canyon walls. A very brief climb through a boulder field leads to a junction ▶4 with the **River Trail** near a bridge across the river.

Fishing

Great Views

Turn right, cross the bridge, and follow gently ascending trail through dense forest and lush groundcover to the day-use parking lot. ▶5

	MILESTONES	
▶1	0.0	Start at trailhead
▶2	1.9	Right at Paradise Valley Trail junction
▶3	2.0	Right at Kanawyer Trail junction
▶4	4.5	Right at River Trail junction
▶5	4.7	End at parking area

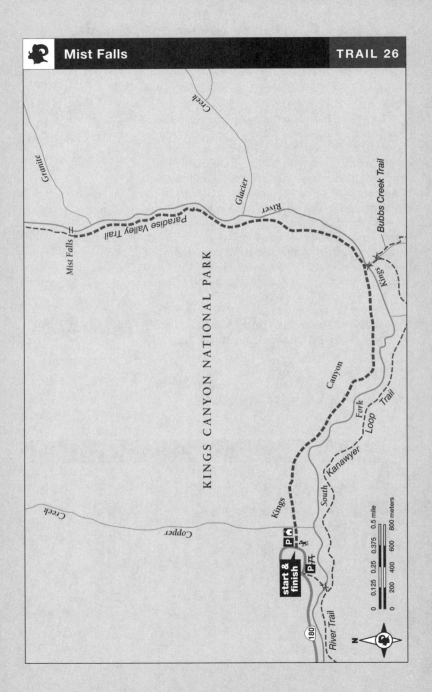

Mist Falls

TRAIL 26

Creek

Granite

Glacier

Creek

River

Bubbs Creek Trail

Paradise Valley Trail

Mist Falls

Kings

KINGS CANYON NATIONAL PARK

Canyon

Fork

Loop Trail

Kanawyer

South

Creek

Copper

Kings

start & finish

180

River Trail

N

0   0.125 0.25 0.375 0.5 mile

0   200   400   600   800 meters

Mist Falls

The nearly 4-mile trek to Mist Falls is a must-do hike for anyone visiting Kings Canyon, especially early in the season when the falls are at peak glory. The first half of the trail follows the relatively flat floor of Kings Canyon, with the second half climbing moderately up the South Fork Kings River gorge toward Paradise Valley. The trail is a popular one, not only with dayhikers, but also with backpackers on the Rae Lakes Loop. Consequently, you shouldn't expect a high dose of solitude.

Best Time

The falls are best appreciated in late spring and early summer, when South Fork Kings River is swollen with snowmelt. By midsummer the falls become fairly tame.

Finding the Trail

From Fresno, follow Highway 180 east into Kings Canyon National Park and continue past Grant Grove into Kings Canyon. Continue up-canyon to the day-use parking area at Roads End, 5.0 miles east of the turnoff to Cedar Grove. The Park Service has four campgrounds in the Cedar Grove area: Sentinel, Sheep Creek, Canyon View, and Moraine (all of which have fees, flush toilets, running water, and bear boxes). Cedar Grove has a motel, showers, general store, restaurant, and laundry facilities.

TRAIL USE
Dayhike, Run, Horse

LENGTH
7.8 miles, 4 hours

VERTICAL FEET
+775/±1550

DIFFICULTY
– 1 2 **3** 4 5 +

TRAIL TYPE
Out & Back

FEATURES
Canyon
Stream
Waterfall
Fishing

FACILITIES
Lodging
Store
Visitors Center
Post Office
Restrooms
Water
Picnic Area
Campgrounds
Stables

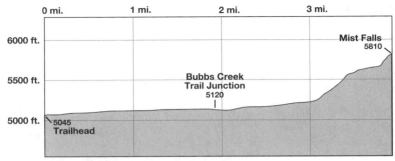

0 mi. 1 mi. 2 mi. 3 mi.

6000 ft.

Mist Falls
5810

5500 ft.

Bubbs Creek
Trail Junction
5120

5000 ft. 5045
Trailhead

TRAIL 26   Mist Falls Elevation Profile

Trail Description

The aptly named falls tumbles over a precipitous cliff and smashes into boulders and rocks near the base.

From the parking area, walk to the well-signed trailhead ▶1 at the east end of the paved turnaround at Roads End, near the rustic cabin that serves as the wilderness permit office. Follow a wide, sandy, gently ascending path that parallels the river through a mixed forest of incense cedars, ponderosa pines, black oaks, sugar pines, and white firs to a bridge across **Copper Creek**. Continue up-canyon into thinning forest cover, which allows occasional views of the impressive granite walls of Kings Canyon, which are often compared favorably to the more famous walls of Yosemite Valley. Soon you enter a shady forest of ponderosa pines, sugar pines, white firs, and alders on the way to a Y-junction with the **Bubbs Creek Trail**. ▶2

Veer left at the junction and follow ascending trail through a mixed forest of alders, black oaks, canyon live oaks, incense cedars, ponderosa pines, and white firs. Occasional clearings in the forest are carpeted with manzanita and mountain mahogany, while ferns and thimbleberries thrive in damper soils. The trail follows the course of the river past delightful pools and tumbling cascades, arcing around the base of Beck Peak. Angers can work their way down to the bank and ply the waters for rainbow and brown trout. Beck, Sphinx, and Avalanche

Fishing

peaks play hide and seek through gaps in the forest cover. Ascending over rock steps and slabs, continue up the narrow chasm of the canyon with occasional views of the dramatic canyon topography. Following a long, forested stretch of trail, the thundering roar from Mist Falls becomes progressively louder the farther up the trail you travel. Soon a use trail splits away from the Paradise Valley Trail to the right and leads over large boulders to a viewpoint near the base of **Mist Falls**. ▶3

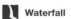 **Waterfall**

The aptly named falls tumbles over a precipitous cliff and smashes into boulders and rocks near the base, creating a spray of mist that catapults down-canyon and coats everything in its path. Even on hot summer days, you can feel cool and moist below the falls, an attribute that must certainly add to this destination's popularity.

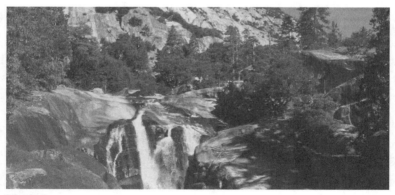

Mist Falls

🚶	MILESTONES	
▶1	0.0	Start at trailhead
▶2	1.9	Left at junction
▶3	3.9	Mist Falls

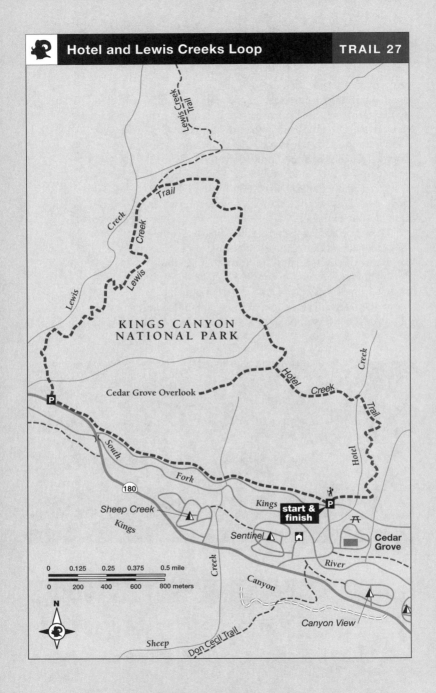

KINGS CANYON
NATIONAL PARK

Lewis Creek Trail

Creek

Creek Trail

Lewis

Lewis

Lewis

P

Cedar Grove Overlook

Hotel Creek

Creek

Hotel Trail

Hotel

P

South Fork

180

Sheep Creek

Kings

Kings

Sentinel

start & finish

P

Cedar Grove

Canyon View

Creek

Canyon

River

Don Cecil Trail

Sheep

| 0 | 0.125 | 0.25 | 0.375 | 0.5 mile |
| 0 | 200 | 400 | 600 | 800 meters |

N

Hotel and Lewis Creeks Loop

Trail users on this loop have the opportunity to sample the transition zones among the riparian woodland community along the banks of South Fork Kings River, foothill woodland on the lower slopes of Kings Canyon, and the mixed coniferous forest and chaparral communities of the canyon rim. Additional interesting ecology is available along the upper part of the loop, where stages of forest succession can be observed following a series of fires that swept through the area. Throw in some great views of Kings Canyon and the Monarch Divide, and the trip has the makings of a fine adventure.

Best Time

Snow usually leaves the trail by sometime in early May and generally doesn't return until November. Since the trail is located on a south-facing slope, an early start to beat the heat will be appreciated on the stiff climb out of Kings Canyon.

Finding the Trail

From Fresno, follow Highway 180 east into Kings Canyon National Park and continue past Grant Grove into Kings Canyon. Continue up-canyon to the signed turnoff to Cedar Grove, turn left and follow signs for the pack station. At 0.5 mile from the highway, turn right and immediately come to the Hotel Creek Trailhead on the left. If you have the luxury of two vehicles, or can arrange for someone to pick you up, 1.4 miles of uninteresting hiking can be saved by ending the trip at the Lewis

TRAIL USE
Dayhike, Run, Horse
LENGTH
6.4 miles, 3–4 hours
VERTICAL FEET
+2475/-2475/±3975
DIFFICULTY
– 1 2 3 **4** 5 +
TRAIL TYPE
Loop

FEATURES
Canyon
Stream
Wildflowers
Great Views

FACILITIES
Lodging
Store
Visitors Center
Post Office
Restrooms
Water
Picnic Area
Campgrounds
Stables

181

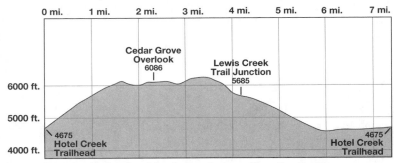

TRAIL 27 Hotel and Lewis Creeks Loop Elevation Profile

Creek Trailhead, which is on the north shoulder of Highway 180 (0.4 mile east of the park boundary and 1.3 miles west of the Cedar Grove junction). The Park Service has four campgrounds in the Cedar Grove area: Sentinel, Sheep Creek, Canyon View, and Moraine (all of which have fees, flush toilets, running water, and bear boxes). Cedar Grove has a motel, showers, general store, restaurant, and laundry facilities.

Trail Description

▶1 Follow the Hotel Creek Trail up a hillside to a junction with a lateral from the pack station. Continue the ascent on the main trail through a mixed forest of oaks, pines, and firs, soon hearing the roar of the creek ahead. Reach the west bank of **Hotel Creek**, where a short use trail heads down to the water's edge, a convenient spot from which to filter water for the stiff and exposed climb above. The trail veers away from the creek and attacks the hillside on a series of switchbacks up the north wall of Kings Canyon. The first half mile offers filtered shade from scattered oaks and pines before the trees are left behind, and you continue the stiff ascent across open, chaparral-covered slopes. The switchbacks eventually end, where the trail veers west away from the creek and the steep ascent is mercifully replaced by a mild to moderate climb that leads to a junction ►2 with a trail on the left to **Cedar Grove Overlook**.

A half-mile detour from the loop route allows you to enjoy a supreme view of Kings Canyon and the Monarch Divide. Turn left (west) at the junction and gently descend through scattered pines with views to the north of Monarch Divide. After a quarter mile, you reach a low spot on a ridge and then begin a mild, short climb toward the overlook, ►3 a knob of granite near the end of a ridge. From this aerie, you gaze spellbound straight down 1500 feet to Cedar Grove at the bottom of Kings Canyon. The bird's-eye view of South Fork Kings River is expansive, spanning from the western foothills to the confluence of Bubbs Creek. To the north, peaks of the Monarch Divide are quite impressive as well. After fully appreciating the view, retrace your steps to the junction.

Turn left at the overlook junction and proceed generally north on a mild descent through a forest of scattered Jeffrey pines that was previously burned and is now carpeted with mountain misery. Lupine and paintbrush add a splash of color in early season. After crossing a couple of seasonal drainages, a moderate climb leads to the high point of the trip on the top of a ridge. Along the way are good views of the Monarch Divide. From the ridgetop, the long descent back to Kings Canyon begins, proceeding through light forest and paralleling an unnamed tributary of Lewis Creek on the way to a junction ►4 with the **Lewis Creek Trail**.

 Wildflowers

 Great Views

Turn left (southwest) at the junction and head downhill through Jeffrey pines in various stages of succession due to the fires common to the area. High above Lewis Creek, you follow numerous switchbacks down-canyon, alternating between brief sections of shade from a mixed forest and

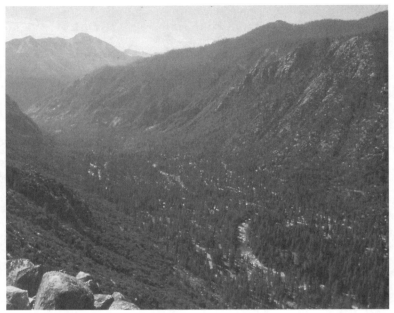

Kings Canyon *from Cedar Grove Overlook*

sunny stretches of chaparral. The protracted descent ends at the **Lewis Creek Trailhead**. ►5

Without the benefit of a second vehicle or someone to pick you up, you must walk southeast from the trailhead on a section of seldom-used trail that parallels the road toward Cedar Grove Village. The 1.4-mile trail seems to needlessly undulate across the hillside above the nearly level road, but the trail does provide a straightforward return route to the **Hotel Creek Trailhead**. ►6

🚶	MILESTONES	
►1	0.0	Start at Hotel Creek Trailhead
►2	1.9	Left at overlook junction
►3	2.3	Cedar Grove Overlook
►4	2.7	Left at overlook junction
►5	4.2	Left at Lewis Creek Trail junction
►6	6.4	Hotel Creek Trailhead

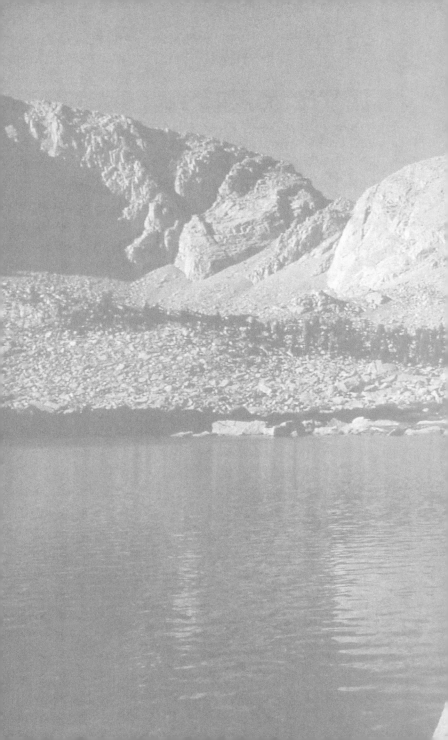

CHAPTER 3

Golden Trout Wilderness, John Muir Wilderness, and East Sequoia

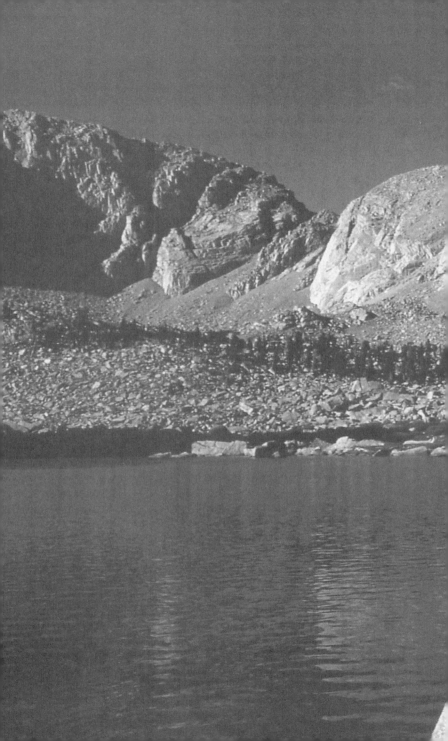

Golden Trout Wilderness, John Muir Wilderness, and East Sequoia

I n sharp contrast to the gently rising western side of the Sierra, the east side rapidly thrusts up from the floor of Owens Valley to form the apex of the High Sierra, a seemingly impenetrable wall of serrated peaks thousands of feet above the valley that would appear to bar all westward penetration. Trails in this region generally take one of two forms: Many paths make no attempt to conquer the crest, instead following raucous streams that terminate in steep, dead-end canyons. A few other paths actually climb over the towering east face of the Sierra on stiff, protracted ascents topping out at passes over 11,000 or 12,000 feet high. Along this section of the Sierra's spine, at 14,494 feet, is the highest point in the continental U.S.—the highly coveted summit of **Mt. Whitney**. A handful of other peaks in the area exceed 14,000 feet, with several more well over 13,000 feet. With such high altitudes and steep topography, hikers and backpackers must not only be well acclimatized but in good physical shape as well.

The high and rugged terrain along the eastern boundary of Sequoia National Park limits the number of Sierra Crest crossings via maintained trail to four: **Cottonwood Pass**, **New Army Pass**, **Trail Crest**, and **Shepherd Pass**. Consequently, available wilderness permits for backpackers desiring to enter the park from the east are oftentimes hard to come by. Demand for the 100 day and 60 overnight permits for the **Mt. Whitney Trail** is so competitive that hikers must enter a lottery for them. With the exception of the Mt. Whitney Trail, day trips into **Golden Trout, John Muir**, and **Sequoia areas** are much more easily arranged than backpacks.

Trails 28–31 all start from the Horseshoe Meadow/Cottonwood Lakes trailheads, with the first trip traveling through the Golden Trout Wilderness over Cottonwood Pass to scenic **Chicken Spring Lake**. Trail 29 is a relatively short journey to several beautiful lakes lying in the eastern shadow of

Overleaf and opposite: *Cottonwood Lakes Basin*

the Sierra Crest. The **Soldier Lakes basin**, cradling two picturesque lakes in a dramatic cirque west of New Army Pass and within Sequoia National Park, is the destination of Trail 30. The six **Cottonwood Lakes** accessed by a relatively short trail in Trail 31 offer excellent opportunities for anglers as well as dayhikers, backpackers, and equestrians. Most trails users driving up the Whitney Portal Road are ultimately bound for the summit of Mt. Whitney, as described in Trail 33, but the journey in Trail 32 from the Whitney Portal Campground to **Meysan Lake**, while much less frequently taken, is well worth the time and energy.

Permits

Wilderness permits are required for all overnight stays in the backcountry of Golden Trout Wilderness, John Muir Wilderness, and Sequoia National Park. Trailhead quotas are in effect from May 1 to November 1 for eastside entry into John Muir Wilderness and from the last Friday in June to September 15 into Golden Trout Wilderness. Sixty percent of the daily quota is available by advanced reservation with a $5 per person fee. Reservations can be made up to six months before the start date of a trip by contacting the Wilderness Permit Office by phone (760-873-2483), or with a downloadable application (www.fs/fed.us/r5/inyo), reservations can also be submitted by fax (760-873-2484), or mail (Inyo National Forest, Wilderness Permit Office, 351 Pacu Lane, Bishop, CA 93514). The remaining 40 percent of the daily quota is available as walk-in permits. These free permits can be picked up beginning at 11 AM the day before the start of a trip through close of business the day of departure. All permits can be picked up at the Mono Basin Scenic Area Visitors Center (Lee Vining), Mammoth Ranger Station (Mammoth Lakes), White Mountain Ranger Station (Bishop), or Eastern Sierra InterAgency Visitors Center (Lone Pine).

Both dayhikers and backpackers entering the Whitney Zone from any trailhead in Inyo National Forest must pay a $15 per person fee. Recreationists using the Mt. Whitney Trail from Whitney Portal must apply for a permit through the Mt. Whitney Lottery. Mail (postmarked with a February date) or fax a completed downloadable form with payment to the Wilderness Permit Office. The lottery process begins on February 15, with successful submissions receiving notification within two months. Consult the Inyo National Forest website (www.fs.fed.us/r5/inyo) for more information about the permit process.

Maps

For Golden Trout Wilderness, John Muir Wilderness, and East Sequoia, the USGS 7.5-minute (1:24,000 scale) topographic maps are listed below.

Trails 28–29: *Cirque Peak*
Trail 30: *Cirque Peak* and *Mount Langley*
Trail 31: *Cirque Peak* and *Johnson Peak*
Trail 32: *Mount Whitney*
Trail 33: *Mount Langley*

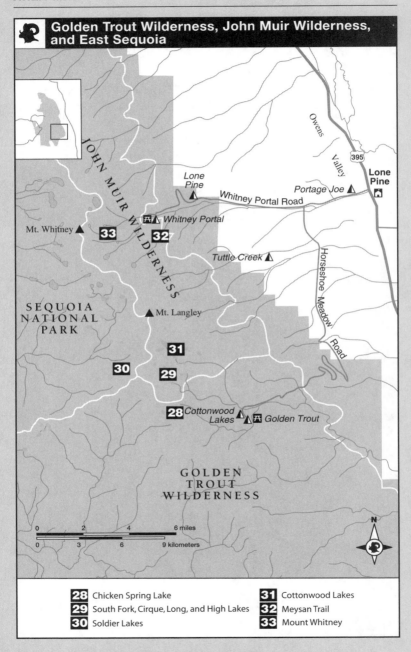

Golden Trout Wilderness, John Muir Wilderness, and East Sequoia

JOHN MUIR WILDERNESS

Owens Valley

395

Lone Pine

Lone Pine ⚑

Portage Joe ▲

Whitney Portal Road

⛺▲ *Whitney Portal*

Mt. Whitney ▲ **33** **32**

Tuttle Creek ▲

Horseshoe Meadow Road

SEQUOIA NATIONAL PARK

▲ Mt. Langley

31

30 **29**

28 *Cottonwood Lakes* ▲ ▲⛺ *Golden Trout*

GOLDEN TROUT WILDERNESS

| 0 | 2 | 4 | 6 miles |
| 0 | 3 | 6 | 9 kilometers |

N

28 Chicken Spring Lake	**31** Cottonwood Lakes
29 South Fork, Cirque, Long, and High Lakes	**32** Meysan Trail
30 Soldier Lakes	**33** Mount Whitney

TRAIL FEATURE TABLE

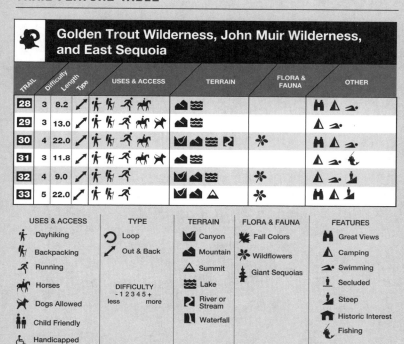

Golden Trout Wilderness, John Muir Wilderness, and East Sequoia

TRAIL	Difficulty	Length	Type	USES & ACCESS	TERRAIN	FLORA & FAUNA	OTHER
28	3	8.2	Out & Back	Dayhiking, Backpacking, Running, Horses	Mountain, Lake		Great Views, Camping, Swimming
29	3	13.0	Out & Back	Dayhiking, Backpacking, Running, Horses, Dogs Allowed	Mountain, Lake		Camping, Swimming
30	4	22.0	Out & Back	Dayhiking, Backpacking, Running, Horses	Canyon, Mountain, Lake, River or Stream	Wildflowers	Great Views, Camping, Swimming
31	3	11.8	Out & Back	Dayhiking, Backpacking, Running, Horses, Dogs Allowed	Mountain, Lake		Camping, Swimming, Fishing
32	4	9.0	Out & Back	Dayhiking, Backpacking, Running	Canyon, Mountain, Lake	Wildflowers	Camping, Swimming, Steep
33	5	22.0	Out & Back	Dayhiking, Backpacking, Running	Canyon, Mountain, Summit	Wildflowers	Great Views, Camping, Steep

USES & ACCESS
- Dayhiking
- Backpacking
- Running
- Horses
- Dogs Allowed
- Child Friendly
- Handicapped Access

TYPE
- Loop
- Out & Back

DIFFICULTY
-1 2 3 4 5 +
less   more

TERRAIN
- Canyon
- Mountain
- Summit
- Lake
- River or Stream
- Waterfall

FLORA & FAUNA
- Fall Colors
- Wildflowers
- Giant Sequoias

FEATURES
- Great Views
- Camping
- Swimming
- Secluded
- Steep
- Historic Interest
- Fishing

Golden Trout Wilderness, John Muir Wilderness, and East Sequoia

Cottonwood Lakes 215

While most eastside High Sierra trails are generally
quite steep, the Cottonwood Lakes is, for the most
part, a pleasant exception, with only about one-
third of the route ascending at a moderate grade.
The relatively easy trail combined with outstanding
scenery and a notable golden-trout fishery make the
area a popular destination for a wide range of recreationists. Despite such popularity, the high number
of lakes in Cottonwood Lakes Basin allows visitors
the opportunity to spread out quite easily.

TRAIL 31

Dayhike, Backpack,
Run, Horse,
Dogs Allowed
11.8 miles, Out & Back
Difficulty: 3

Meysan Trail 221

While hundreds toil along the nearby Mt. Whitney
Trail, a relative few hike this neighboring path up
the canyon of Meysan Creek to a string of attractive
lakes east of the Sierra Crest.

TRAIL 32

Dayhike, Backpack, Run
9.0 miles, Out & Back
Difficulty: 4

Mount Whitney 225

Despite the hassle of entering the lottery and angling
for a permit with far too many Whitney pilgrims,
hiking the 11-mile trail to the summit of the Lower
48's loftiest summit remains one of the High Sierra's
most epic adventures and most notable achieve-
ments. The view from the summit is sublime, but
the scenery along the way is as equally rewarding.

TRAIL 33

Dayhike, Backpack, Run
22.0 miles, Out & Back
Difficulty: 5

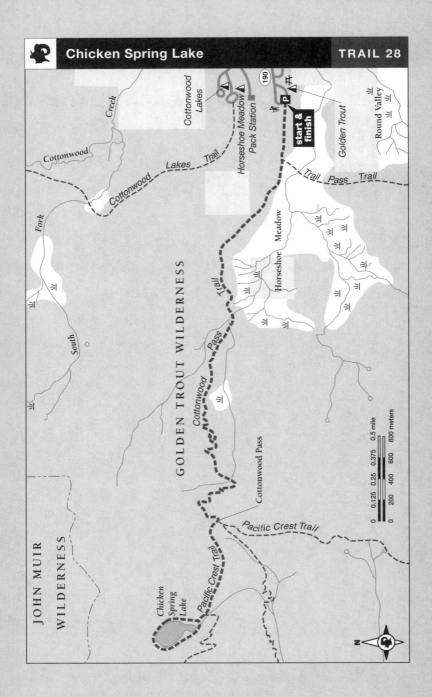

Chicken Spring Lake

TRAIL 28

190

Cottonwood Creek

Cottonwood Lakes

Horseshoe Meadow Pack Station

start & finish

P

Golden Trout

Round Valley

Cottonwood

Cottonwood Lakes Trail

Trail Pass Trail

Fork

Horseshoe Meadow

South

GOLDEN TROUT WILDERNESS

Cottonwood Pass Trail

Cottonwood Pass

Pacific Crest Trail

JOHN MUIR WILDERNESS

Chicken Spring Lake

Pacific Crest Trail

N

0   0.125   0.25   0.375   0.5 mile

0   200   400   600   800 meters

Chicken Spring Lake

Aside from a 0.75-mile switchbacking climb to an 11,000-foot pass, the grade of the trail is gentle, offering recreationists a relatively easy 4-plus-mile trip to scenic Chicken Spring Lake. Views along the way from Cottonwood Pass of the Great Western Divide to the west and the Panamint and Inyo mountains to the east are quite scenic. Although the trail is straightforward and the distance is short, the lake sees far fewer visitors than expected, helping to make this a fine destination for hikers, backpackers, anglers, and swimmers.

Best Time

With a location in the High Sierra, trails are usually snow-free by mid-July and remain so through mid-October.

Finding the Trail

In the town of Lone Pine, turn west from U.S. Highway 395 and follow Whitney Portal Road for 3 miles to a left-hand turn onto Horseshoe Meadow Road. Head south for 18.5 miles, passing the turnoff to Cottonwood Lakes, to the Horseshoe Meadows parking lot at the end of the road. The trailhead has vault toilets, running water, and a walk-in campground nearby (one-night limit, fee, vault toilets, running water, bear boxes, and phone).

TRAIL USE
Dayhike, Backpack, Run, Horse
LENGTH
8.2 miles, 4 hours
VERTICAL FEET
+1400/-100/±3000
DIFFICULTY
– 1 2 **3** 4 5 +
TRAIL TYPE
Out & Back

FEATURES
Mountain
Lake
Great Views
Camping
Swimming

FACILITIES
Campground
Picnic Area
Stables

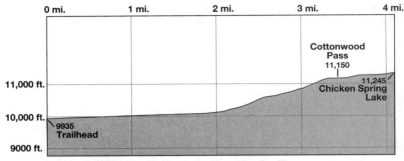

TRAIL 28   Chicken Spring Lake Elevation Profile

Logistics

Backpackers must obtain a wilderness permit for all overnight visits. See page 190 for more details about how to obtain one.

Trail Description

►1 The well-signed trail begins by an interpretive signboard near the restrooms and follows gently graded, wide, and sandy tread through scattered lodgepole and foxtail pines. The sandy soil is nearly barren of ground cover. Shortly cross the **Golden Trout Wilderness boundary** and reach a junction ►2 with trails heading south to Trail Pass and north to the pack station. Continue ahead (west) from the junction along the fringe of expansive **Horseshoe Meadow** on nearly level and sandy tread that may remind you of trudging through beach sand. Where the forest thickens, come alongside and then across a stream. On the far bank, a use trail leads to the remains of a dilapidated cabin (no camping). The trail shortly crosses back over the stream, leaves Horseshoe Meadow behind, and then begins a moderate ascent. Farther along, a series of switchbacks leads up a rock-strewn hillside along a willow-lined drainage, eventually zigzagging up to 11,200-foot **Cottonwood Pass**. The fine view includes

The shoreline is peppered with foxtail pines, with several weather-beaten snags adding a little character to the picture-postcard scene.

Horseshoe Meadow backdropped picturesquely by the Panamint and Inyo mountains to the east and the southern tip of the Great Western Divide to the west. A very short distance beyond the pass is a junction ▶3 with the **Pacific Crest Trail** and a path heading southwest toward Big Whitney Meadow.

 Great Views

Following a sign toward Rock Creek, you turn right on the PCT to proceed northwest on an easy half-mile traverse to Chicken Spring Lake's seasonal outlet and a use-trail junction. ▶4 Leave the PCT here and follow the use trail upstream to the south shore of the lake. ▶5

 Lake

Tucked into a cirque bowl, **Chicken Spring Lake** is nearly surrounded by rugged granite cliffs. The shoreline is peppered with foxtail pines, with several weather-beaten snags adding a little character to the picture-postcard scene. Several good campsites (no fires) occupy sandy patches around a small bay on the south side near the outlet, and in scattered pines above the west shore. A use trail nearly encircles the shoreline, providing access to the cool waters for both anglers and swimmers.

 Camping

🚶	**MILESTONES**	
▶1	0.0	Start at trailhead
▶2	0.35	Straight at junction
▶3	3.4	Right on Pacific Crest Trail
▶4	4.0	Right at use trail
▶5	4.1	Chicken Spring Lake

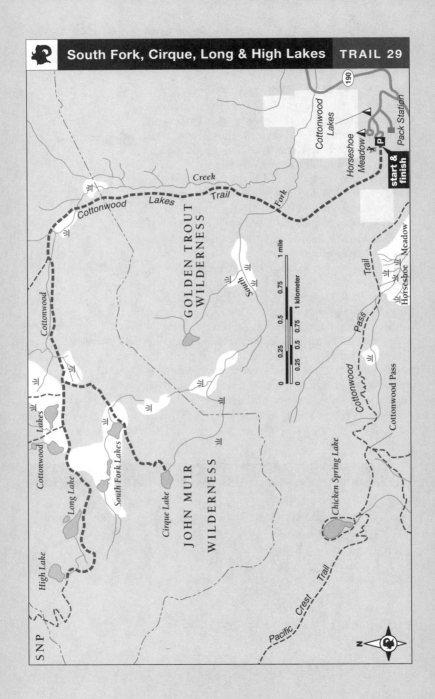

190

Cottonwood Lakes

Pack Station

Horseshoe Meadow

P

start & finish

Creek

Cottonwood   Lakes   Trail

Fork

Horseshoe Meadow

GOLDEN TROUT WILDERNESS

South

Horseshoe Pass Trail

Cottonwood

1 mile

0.75

0.5

1 kilometer

0.25   0.5   0.75

0   0.25   0.5

0

Cottonwood Pass Trail

Cottonwood Pass

Cottonwood Lakes

Long Lake

South Fork Lakes

Cirque Lake

JOHN MUIR WILDERNESS

Chicken Spring Lake

High Lake

Pacific   Crest   Trail

S N P

N

South Fork, Cirque, Long, and High Lakes

The gently graded trails into this area provide a reasonably easy trip to a handful of scenic lakes along the New Army Pass and South Fork Lakes trails, where a plethora of open, rock-strewn basins and grassy meadows permit fine views of the rugged eastern Sierra Crest. Although this picturesque area is quite popular during the height of summer, many of the more far-flung lakes are lightly visited.

Best Time

Snow leaves the area by mid-July following an average winter, and the typically sunny and mild Sierra weather continues through summer. Autumn can be a pleasant time for a hike because the crowds diminish and the weather is cooler but generally sunny. The first significant snowfall at these elevations usually comes sometime by late October or early November.

Finding the Trail

In the town of Lone Pine, turn west from U.S. Highway 395 and follow Whitney Portal Road for 3 miles to a left-hand turn onto Horseshoe Meadow Road. Head south for 18.5 miles, and turn right toward Cottonwood Lakes. Pass the Cottonwood Lakes walk-in campground (one-night limit, fee, vault toilets, running water, bear boxes, and phone) and continue to the trailhead parking area, 0.5 mile from Horseshoe Meadows Road. The trailhead has vault toilets and running water.

TRAIL USE
Dayhike, Backpack, Run, Horse, Dogs Allowed

LENGTH
13.0 miles, 7 hours

VERTICAL FEET
+1650/-235/±3770

DIFFICULTY
− 1 2 **3** 4 5 +

TRAIL TYPE
Out & Back

FEATURES
Mountain
Lake
Camping
Swimming

FACILITIES
Campground
Picnic Area
Stables

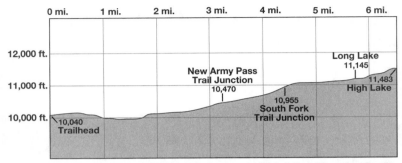

TRAIL 29   South Fork, Cirque, Long, and High Lakes Elevation Profile

Logistics

Backpackers must obtain a wilderness permit for all overnight visits. See page 190 for more details about how to obtain one.

Trail Description

►1 The Cottonwood Lakes Trail begins somewhat auspiciously as a short, brick-lined path near a restroom building and a trailhead signboard. Sandy tread leads away from the trailhead on a gentle ascent through widely scattered foxtail and lodgepole pines, where virtually no ground cover is able to take root in the sandy soil. Soon cross into **Golden Trout Wilderness** and pass a spur trail on the left headed toward the pack station. ►2 From there, an equally gentle ascent leads down to a crossing of South Fork Cottonwood Creek, 1 mile from the trailhead, where a few campsites are found on the far bank. The lush vegetation along the banks of the creek seems especially vibrant after the dearth of plant life in the first mile.

From the creek, the trail climbs gently through more scattered pines to the main branch of **Cottonwood Creek** and then follows this stream up a broad valley for the next 1.5 miles. Along

Camping

South Fork and Cirque Lakes

A side trip to these lakes is a fine diversion for those with the extra time and energy. From the junction, head south along the fringe of a sloping meadow lined with willows and then veer southwest on a gentle climb through foxtail pines. A short descent leads to a crossing of South Fork Cottonwood Creek, and then the trail slices across a large meadow to the east side of the easternmost South Fork Lake. The roughly oval-shaped lake, splendidly backdropped by rocky ridges and craggy peaks, offers backpackers a few choice campsites on a hill above the southwest shore. A straightforward cross-country jaunt leads to the upper South Fork Lakes.

To visit Cirque Lake, follow the continuation of the trail on a moderate climb through scattered foxtail pines to the apex of a ridge and then descend shortly to the northeast shore. The lake has a decidedly alpine ambiance, nestled at the base of steep cliffs below the rugged profile of Cirque Peak. A few campsites are scattered around the sparsely forested shoreline, but the number seems more than adequate for the few adventurous souls who travel this far off the Cottonwood Lakes and New Army Pass trails.

the way, you cross the boundary separating the Golden Trout and John Muir wilderness areas, in the shadow of steep rock cliffs on the left and within view of the wood structures of Golden Trout Camp across a meadow on the right. Beyond the boundary, the trail veers west on a more moderate ascent up the narrowing canyon. At 2.5 miles, cross the creek on a beveled log and pass more campsites near the meadow-lined stream. Just after the crossing of a side stream is a junction of the **Cottonwood Lakes and New Army Pass trails**. ▶3

Camping

Leaving the Cottonwood Lakes Trail, you veer left at the junction, soon cross to the south side of Cottonwood Creek, and then climb moderately for a little over a mile to a junction with South Fork Lakes Trail beside a large meadow. ▶4

To continue toward Cottonwood Lakes, proceed ahead (west) at the **South Fork Lakes Trail**

Cottonwood Lakes

Backpackers blessed with an extra day or two can easily journey to the neighboring Cottonwood Lakes, as described in Trail 31 (see page 215). The relatively easy travel combined with outstanding scenery and a noteworthy golden-trout fishery makes the area quite popular with a wide range of outdoor enthusiasts. However, solitude seekers should not despair, as the bounty of lakes tends to disperse visitors around the basin. The extensive network of trails and easy cross-country jaunts makes travel from one lake to another fairly easy. Anglers should stay abreast of fishing regulations, which limit Lakes 1–4 to catch and release only. All lakes in the basin are restricted to artificial lures or flies with barbless hooks, with a limit of five fish.

junction and make a short climb up a hillside to a Y-junction with a connector to the Cottonwood Lakes Trail. ►5 Keep heading west on the **New Army Pass Trail,** skirting the edge of a large meadow surrounding **Cottonwood Lake 1** and continuing past **Lake 2.** Leaving the meadowland behind, make a short climb to a desolate area filled with scads of large granite boulders, where only a few scattered pockets of pines seem able to gain a foothold in this sea of rock. Eventually the boulders are left behind as gently graded trail arcs around a lightly forested hillside. Below, a meadow-lined, refreshing-looking stream rushes toward the westernmost South Fork Lake. A faint use trail leads across the stream to forested campsites between this lake and Long Lake above. A more moderate climb then leads up through thinning forest to the south shore of **Long Lake,** ►6 where the best campsites are found beneath a stand of pines near the southwest shore, with a few less protected sites above the north shore.

Lake

Camping

From the east shore of Long Lake, the New Army Pass Trail climbs steeper toward **High Lake** and the pass beyond. Through grasses, low-growing alpine plants, and widely scattered, dwarf pines, you climb to timberline and then wind up rocky switchbacks to High Lake. ▶7 The lake is set in a rocky, open bowl rimmed by steep cliffs, the rocky terrain severely limiting the opportunity for decent campsites. For those interested in additional pursuits, the moderately graded mile climb to **New Army Pass** at the boundary of Sequoia National Park offers wide-ranging views.

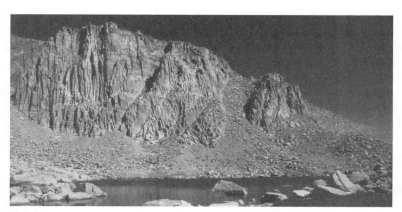

High Lake

六	MILESTONES	
▶1	0.0	Start at trailhead
▶2	0.1	Ahead at pack station spur
▶3	3.25	Left at New Army Pass Trail junction
▶4	4.4	Ahead at South Fork Lakes Trail junction
▶5	4.5	Ahead at connector junction
▶6	5.75	Long Lake
▶7	6.5	High Lake

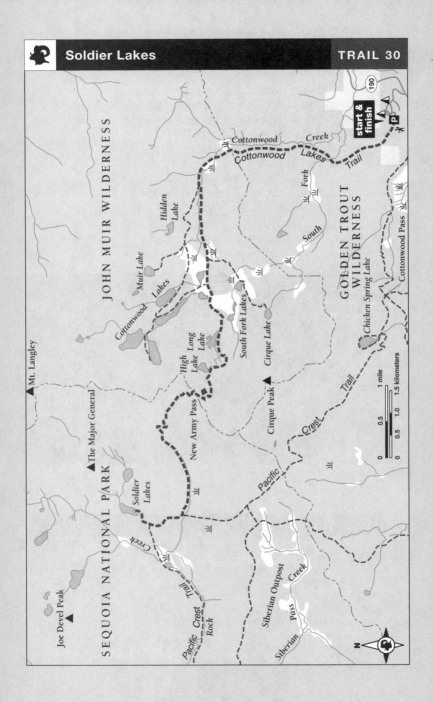

190

start & finish

P

Cottonwood *Creek*

Cottonwood Lakes Trail

JOHN MUIR WILDERNESS

Hidden Lake

South Fork

GOLDEN TROUT WILDERNESS

Muir Lake

Cottonwood Lakes

Chicken Spring Lake

Cottonwood Pass

Mt. Langley

High Long Lake Lake

South Fork Lakes

Cirque Lake

Cirque Peak

The Major General

New Army Pass

Pacific Crest Trail

SEQUOIA NATIONAL PARK

Soldier Lakes

1 mile

1.5 kilometers

0.5   1.0

0   0.5

Joe Devel Peak

Pacific Crest Rock

Creek Trail

Siberian Outpost

Siberian Creek

Siberian Pass

N

Soldier Lakes

Strong hikers may be able to cover the entire 22-mile distance to Lower Soldier Lake and back, but this trip is perhaps better suited to backpackers with at least a weekend to fully enjoy the marvelous scenery. Most visitors to the area are content with destinations in the Cottonwood Lakes Basin, but some truly wonderful terrain lies on the other side of New Army Pass, including the two Soldier Lakes majestically backdropped by the towering slopes of the Major General. Along the way, wildflower-carpeted meadows, a delightful stream, and serene forests (not to mention the fine view from New Army Pass) will gladden the heart.

Best Time

Snow leaves the area by mid-July following an average winter and the typically sunny and mild Sierra weather continues through summer. Autumn can be a pleasant time for a hike because the crowds diminish and the weather is cooler but generally sunny. The first significant snowfall at these elevations usually comes sometime by late October or early November.

Finding the Trail

In the town of Lone Pine, turn west from U.S. Highway 395 and follow Whitney Portal Road for 3 miles to a left-hand turn onto Horseshoe Meadow Road. Head south for 18.5 miles, and turn right toward Cottonwood Lakes. Pass the Cottonwood Lakes walk-in campground (one-night limit, fee,

TRAIL USE
Dayhike, Backpack,
Run, Horse
LENGTH
22.0 miles, 11–12 hours
VERTICAL FEET
+2425/-1700/±8250
DIFFICULTY
– 1 2 3 **4** 5 +
TRAIL TYPE
Out & Back

FEATURES
Canyon
Mountain
Lake
Stream
Wildflowers
Great Views
Camping
Swimming

FACILITIES
Campground
Picnic Area
Stables

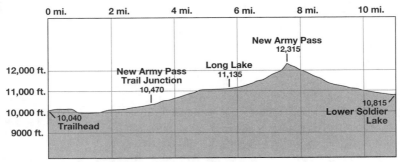

TRAIL 30 Soldier Lakes Elevation Profile

vault toilets, running water, bear boxes, and phone)
and continue to the trailhead parking area, 0.5 mile
from Horseshoe Meadow Road. The trailhead has
vault toilets and running water.

Logistics

Backpackers must obtain a wilderness permit for all
overnight visits. See page 190 for more details about
how to obtain one.

Trail Description

►1 The Cottonwood Lakes Trail begins somewhat
auspiciously as a short, brick-lined path near a
restroom building and a trailhead signboard. Sandy
tread leads away from the trailhead on a gentle
ascent through widely scattered foxtail and lodgepole pines, where virtually no ground cover is able
to take root in the sandy soil. Soon you cross into
Golden Trout Wilderness and pass a spur trail on
the left headed toward the pack station. ►2 From
there, an equally gentle grade leads down to a crossing of South Fork Cottonwood Creek, 1 mile from
the trailhead, where a few campsites are found on
the far bank. The lush vegetation along the banks of

Camping

the creek seems especially vibrant after the dearth of plant life in the first mile.

From the creek, the trail climbs gently through more scattered pines to the main branch of Cottonwood Creek and then follows this stream up a broad valley for the next 1.5 miles. Along the way, you cross the boundary separating the Golden Trout and John Muir wilderness areas, in the shadow of steep rock cliffs on the left and within view of the wood structures of Golden Trout Camp across a meadow on the right. Beyond the boundary, the trail veers west on a more moderate ascent up the narrowing canyon. At 2.5 miles, cross the creek on a beveled log and pass more campsites near the meadow-lined stream. Just after the crossing of a side stream is a junction of the **Cottonwood Lakes and New Army Pass trails**. ▶3

Wildflowers

Leaving the Cottonwood Lakes Trail, you veer left at the junction, soon cross to the south side of Cottonwood Creek, and then climb moderately for a little over a mile to a junction with **South Fork Lakes Trail** beside a large meadow. ▶4

Continuing toward Cottonwood Lakes, proceed ahead (west) at the South Fork Lakes Trail junction and make a short climb up a hillside to a Y-junction with a connector to the Cottonwood Lakes Trail. ▶5 Keep heading west on the New Army Pass Trail, skirting the edge of a large meadow surrounding **Cottonwood Lake 1** and continuing past **Lake 2**. Leaving the meadowland behind, make a short climb to a desolate area filled with scads of large granite boulders, where only a few scattered pockets of pines seem able to gain a foothold in this sea of rock. Eventually the boulders are left behind as gently graded trail arcs around a lightly forested hillside. Below, a meadow-lined, refreshing-looking stream rushes toward the westernmost South Fork Lake. A faint use trail leads across the stream to forested campsites between this lake and Long Lake above.

Army and New Army Passes

Army Pass, a little less than a half mile north of New Army Pass, was the route of the original trail built in 1892. Oversight of Sequoia National Park at that time was the responsibility of the U.S. Army and a contingent of African-Americans from Georgia was assigned the task of improving a trail over the Sierra Crest originally used by sheepherders. The trail was rerouted to cross New Army Pass in 1955, as Army Pass was notorious for hanging onto snowfields well into summer.

 Lake

 Camping

A more moderate climb then leads up through thinning forest to the south shore of **Long Lake**, ▶6 where the best campsites are found beneath a stand of pines near the southwest shore, with a few less-protected sites above the north shore.

From the east shore of Long Lake, the New Army Pass Trail climbs steeper toward High Lake and the pass beyond. Through grasses, low-growing alpine plants, and widely scattered, dwarf pines, you climb to timberline and then wind up rocky switchbacks to **High Lake**. ▶7 The lake is set in a rocky, open bowl rimmed by steep cliffs, the rocky terrain severely limiting the opportunity for decent campsites.

From High Lake, rocky switchbacks lead up to **New Army Pass**. ▶8

Great Views

After enjoying the wide-ranging view from the pass, descend barren slopes to more hospitable terrain below, where you eventually meet and then follow a tributary of Rock Creek through boulder-sprinkled meadows below rocky cliffs and ridges. Stunted pines make an appearance, followed by flower-filled meadows beneath a scattered to light forest of lodgepole and foxtail pines on the way to a junction ▶9 with a lateral heading south to the Pacific Crest Trail.

Veer right at the lateral junction and pass a thin strip of meadow on the way to a signed lateral ▶10 leading to pine-shaded campsites with a bear box on a low rise above the outlet from Soldier Lakes. Continue ahead a short distance to a boulder-hop of the outlet and a junction on the far side with the trail to Soldier Lakes. ▶11

Turn right and head northeast from the junction to follow the edge of a narrow, flower-filled meadow beneath scattered pines to the southern tip of the lower lake. Although a boot-beaten path continues along the west shore, the best campsites are nestled under pines on a rise above the southeast shore. Work your way over to the outlet just below the lake and make the crossing on some well-placed logs and rocks. Once on the far side, follow a faint path along the southeast shore to the camping area on the southeast side of **Lower Soldier Lake**. ▶12 Dramatically framed by the towering walls of the Major General, Lower Soldier Lake reposes in a scenic cirque. Anglers should enjoy fishing for the resident golden trout.

 Lake

Upper Soldier Lake and Miter Basin

OPTIONS

Backpackers with plenty of time and off-trail skills can extend their journey on various cross-country routes in the upper Rock Creek drainage. Upper Soldier Lake is an easy jaunt east from the north shore of Lower Rock Lake. A more ambitious route follows Rock Creek by returning to the junction, heading southwest on the New Army Pass Trail for 0.6 mile to the crossing of Rock Creek, and then leaving the trail to follow a use trail north-northeast along the east bank of the creek. The discernible path eventually falters, but the route-finding is straightforward from there to isolated Miter Basin.

⚐ MILESTONES

►1	0.0	Start at trailhead
►2	0.1	Ahead at pack station spur
►3	3.25	Left at New Army Pass Trail junction
►4	4.4	Ahead at South Fork Lakes Trail junction
►5	4.5	Ahead at connector junction
►6	6.5	Long Lake
►7	6.5	High Lake
►8	7.5	New Army Pass
►9	9.9	Right at lateral to Pacific Crest Trail
►10	10.4	Straight at lateral to campsites
►11	10.5	Right at Soldier Lakes Trail
►12	11.0	Lower Soldier Lake

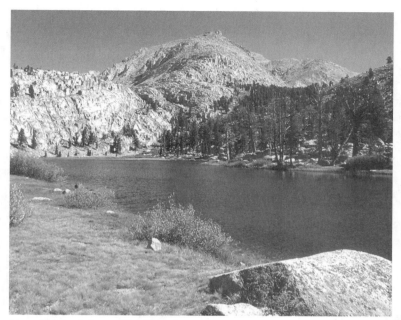

Lower Soldier Lake and the Major General

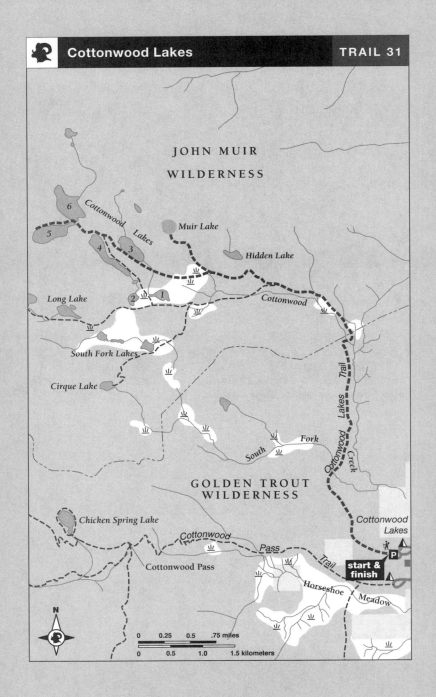

JOHN MUIR

WILDERNESS

Cottonwood
Lakes

6

5

4

3

2

1

Muir Lake

Hidden Lake

Long Lake

Cottonwood

South Fork Lakes

Cirque Lake

South   Fork

Cottonwood   Lakes   Trail

Cottonwood   Creek

GOLDEN TROUT
WILDERNESS

Chicken Spring Lake

Cottonwood

Pass

Cottonwood Pass

Trail

Cottonwood
Lakes

start &
finish

Horseshoe   Meadow

N

0   0.25   0.5   .75 miles

0   0.5   1.0   1.5 kilometers

Cottonwood Lakes

Aside from a 1.75-mile stretch of moderate climbing, the journey to Cottonwood Lakes is on gently graded trail. The relatively easy trail, outstanding scenery, and noted golden trout fishery combine to make this area a popular destination for a wide range of recreationists. Travel between the lakes via a fine network of trails and easy cross-country routes makes getting around fairly straightforward. Solitude seekers should be able to find some secluded spots away from the main thoroughfare.

Best Time

Snow leaves the area by mid-July following an average winter and the typically sunny and mild Sierra weather continues through summer. Autumn can be a pleasant time for a hike because the crowds diminish and the weather is cooler but generally sunny. The first significant snowfall at these elevations usually comes sometime by late October or early November.

Finding the Trail

In the town of Lone Pine, turn west from U.S. Highway 395 and follow Whitney Portal Road for 3 miles to a left-hand turn onto Horseshoe Meadow Road. Head south for 18.5 miles, and turn right toward Cottonwood Lakes. Pass the Cottonwood Lakes walk-in campground (one-night limit, fee, vault toilets, running water, bear boxes, and phone) and continue to the trailhead parking area, 0.5 mile

TRAIL USE
Dayhike, Backpack,
Run, Horse,
Dogs Allowed
LENGTH
11.8 miles, 6 hours
VERTICAL FEET
+1450/-300/±3500
DIFFICULTY
– 1 2 **3** 4 5 +
TRAIL TYPE
Out & Back

FEATURES
Mountain
Lake
Camping
Swimming
Fishing

FACILITIES
Campground
Picnic Area
Stables

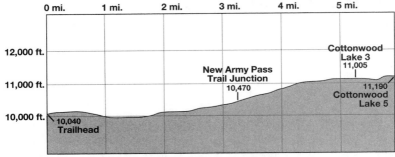

TRAIL 31 Cottonwood Lakes Elevation Profile

from Horseshoe Meadow Road. The trailhead has vault toilets and running water.

Logistics

Backpackers must obtain a wilderness permit for all overnight visits. See page 190 for more details about how to obtain one.

Trail Description

►1 The Cottonwood Lakes Trail begins somewhat auspiciously as a short, brick-lined path near a restroom building and a trailhead signboard. Sandy tread leads away from the trailhead on a gentle ascent through widely scattered foxtail and lodgepole pines, where virtually no ground cover is able to take root in the sandy soil. Soon cross into Golden Trout Wilderness and pass a spur trail on the left headed toward the pack station. ►2 From there, an equally gentle grade leads down to a crossing of South Fork Cottonwood Creek, 1 mile from the trailhead, where a few campsites are found on the far bank. The lush vegetation along the banks of the creek seems especially vibrant after the dearth of plant life in the first mile.

The relatively easy trail, outstanding scenery, and noted golden trout fishery combine to make this area a popular destination for a wide range of recreationists.

 Camping

From the creek, the trail climbs gently through more scattered pines to the main branch of Cottonwood Creek and then follows this stream up a broad valley for the next 1.5 miles. Along the way, you cross the boundary separating the Golden Trout and John Muir wilderness areas, in the shadow of steep rock cliffs on the left and within view of the wood structures of Golden Trout Camp across a meadow on the right. Beyond the boundary, the trail veers west on a more moderate ascent up the narrowing canyon. At 2.5 miles, cross the creek on a beveled log and pass more campsites near the meadow-lined stream. Just after the crossing of a side stream is a junction of the **Cottonwood Lakes and New Army Pass trails**. ▶3

Veer right at the junction and continue up the Cottonwood Lakes Trail on a moderate climb through lodgepole and foxtail pine forest on an

OPTIONS

Muir Lake

Muir Lake makes a fine diversion for those with extra time and energy. The beginning of the trail is somewhat difficult to discern, but the designated route follows a faint path that skirts the northeast side of the meadow and then bends north toward the lake (in spite of some indication that the trail heads northeast up a low hill on the right, which is the beginning of a cross-country route to Hidden Lake). Follow the path around the meadow and then ascend north through pines and scattered boulders to a flower-lined rivulet. From there, continue on a sometimes indistinct path toward the lake, which is hard to miss, despite the periodically disappearing nature of the trail, as the lake is tucked into a horseshoe-shaped cirque at the base of an unnamed peak (3913).

Muir Lake is quite scenic, with rugged cliffs partially encircling the basin and the upper slopes of Mt. Langley towering over the terrain to the northwest. Judging by the condition of the trail, the lake appears to see few visitors, in spite of the pleasant scenery and a selection of fine campsites shaded by scattered pines.

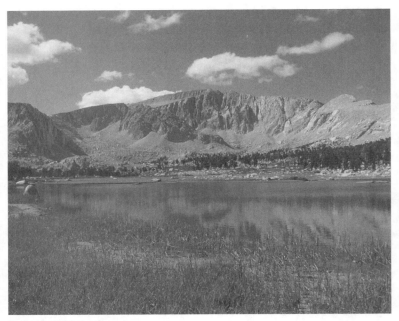

Cottonwood Lake 3

ascent that leads well above the creek to a series of switchbacks. Through the trees you have occasional views up the canyon to Cirque Peak and the east Sierra Crest. At the eastern edge of an expansive meadow, near the lip of the Cottonwood Lakes basin, you reach a signed junction with a lateral to Muir Lake. ▶4

Continue ahead (west) from the Muir Lake junction on gently graded trail well to the right of Cottonwood Lake 1. The trail soon bends northwest up a low, forested rise (campsites), crosses a stream, and then heads across a grassy meadow dotted with boulders, clumps of willow, and widely scattered pines. From the meadow, the massive east wall of the Sierra Crest looms over the surroundings. Pass by a corrugated metal shed on the left and a

▲ Camping

small tarn on the right before arriving at willow-rimmed **Cottonwood Lake 3**. ▶5 Fine campsites on a forested rise between Lakes 3 and 4 will lure overnighters.

From the northwest end of Lake 3 the trail briefly skirts a meadow and then follows a gentle course through mostly open terrain to the north tip of **Lake 4**. Here, indistinct tread marked by a sign simply reading TRAIL, marks a faint path that follows the east shore of Lake 4 southeast for a mile to a junction with the New Army Pass Trail near Lake 1. To visit **Lake 5**, ▶6 head northwest up a steep hillside to a short stretch of creek connecting two large bodies of water, rimmed by steep cliffs and talus piles, and meadows with scattered clumps of willows. A lack of trees leaves the handful of campsites sprinkled around the shoreline exposed to the elements—much better sites can be found on the rise between Lakes 3 and 4. A straightforward, mile-long cross-country jaunt leads to the seldom visited and diminutive upper lake. While golden trout can be found in all the Cottonwood Lakes, the upper lakes are the only ones that are not catch and release. All lakes in Cottonwood Lakes Basin are restricted to artificial lures or flies with barbless hooks and the limit is 5.

🚶	MILESTONES	
▶1	0.0	Start at trailhead
▶2	0.1	Ahead at pack station spur
▶3	3.25	Right at New Army Pass Trail junction
▶4	4.5	Straight at lateral to Muir Lake
▶5	5.25	Cottonwood Lake 3
▶6	5.9	Cottonwood Lake 5

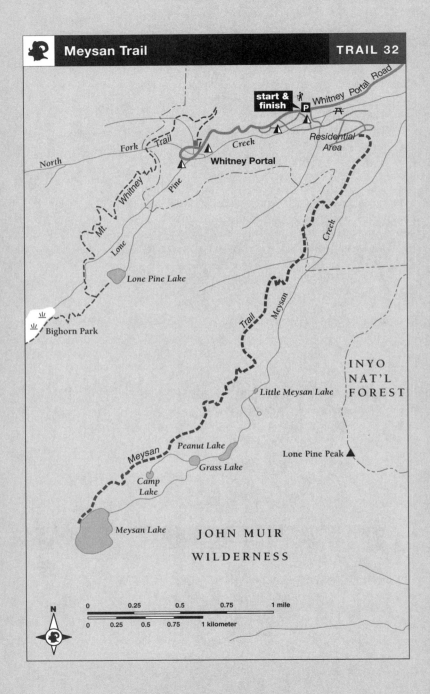

Whitney Portal Road

start & finish

P

Residential Area

North

Fork Trail

Creek

Mt. Whitney

Whitney Portal

Pine

Lone

Lone Pine Lake

Creek

Meysan

Bighorn Park

Trail

INYO NAT'L FOREST

Little Meysan Lake

Meysan

Trail

Peanut Lake

Lone Pine Peak

Grass Lake

Camp Lake

Meysan Lake

JOHN MUIR

WILDERNESS

| 0 | 0.25 | 0.5 | 0.75 | 1 mile |
| 0 | 0.25 | 0.5 | 0.75 | 1 kilometer |

N

Meysan Trail

While hundreds toil along the nearby Mt. Whitney Trail, a relative few hike this neighboring path up the canyon of Meysan Creek to a string of attractive lakes east of the Sierra Crest. Once the typical hubbub of Whitney Portal is left behind, visitors experience quiet serenity on the ascent up Meysan Creek canyon to the end of the trail at Meysan Lake, a fine destination for lunch or for an overnight camp.

Best Time

The Meysan Trail, in the rain shadow of lofty Mt. Whitney, is usually snow-free by early July.

Finding the Trail

From Lone Pine, head west from U.S. Highway 395 on the Whitney Portal Road and drive 13 miles to Whitney Portal, parking your vehicle either in the day-use or overnight parking lots. Campgrounds, a picnic area, restrooms, a store, and a cafe are all nearby. To begin the hike you must descend the old service road from the parking area to the Whitney Portal Campground (fee, flush toilets, running water, bear boxes, and phone). Following a series of signs, walk along the campground loop road across Lone Pine Creek to an intersection. Turn left, pass some summer homes, and make a steep climb to the official trailhead on your right.

TRAIL USE
Dayhike, Backpack, Run

LENGTH
9.0 miles, 5 hours

VERTICAL FEET
+3850/-300/±8300

DIFFICULTY
– 1 2 3 **4** 5 +

TRAIL TYPE
Out & Back

FEATURES
Canyon
Mountain
Lake
Wildflowers
Camping
Swimming
Steep

FACILITIES
Campground
Picnic Area
Store
Cafe
Showers

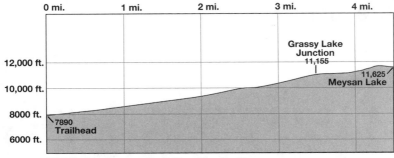

TRAIL 32 Meysan Trail Elevation Profile

Logistics

Backpackers must obtain a wilderness permit for all overnight visits. See page 190 for more details about how to obtain one.

See page 190 for more details about how to obtain one.

Trail Description

At the first of many switchbacks to come, you have good views to the northeast of Alabama Hills and Owens Valley.

▶1 From the official trailhead, follow single-track trail on a steep climb up the hillside. Fortunately, the steep grade is short-lived, as the trail soon merges with another section of road that leads past more summer homes to the resumption of trail.

Having left the last vestiges of civilization behind, you embark on a more moderate climb that leads across a dry hillside dotted with firs, pinyon pines, Jeffrey pines, and mountain mahogany. Soon the trail bends into the canyon of Meysan Creek and curves southwest, slicing across a steep hillside well above the creek. At the first of many switchbacks to come, you have good views to the northeast of Alabama Hills and Owens Valley. Cross into the signed John Muir Wilderness at 1.5 miles.

Continue the switchbacking climb up the canyon, drawing slightly closer to the level of the creek as you go. Along the way is a fine view of a pretty cascade gliding down a rock slab into a delightful pool. More switchbacks lead to even better views farther up the canyon, including another cascade dropping down the headwall of the lake-filled basin above. Scattered foxtail pines start to appear just before a grassy meadow. Nearby a trail sign directs traffic ahead to Grass Lake and to Meysan Lake to the right. ▶2

The tread is a little indistinct beyond the junction, but ducks periodically mark the faint trail on the final climb to Meysan Lake. Bend around a large meadow bordering Camp Lake and then ascend a grassy colouir. Where the slope ahead becomes steeper, veer southwest and climb over rock slabs to a gap above the lake. A short descent from there leads to the northeast shore of Meysan Lake, ▶3 where small pockets of flower-filled meadows dot the otherwise rocky shore and the dramatic headwall formed by Mts. Irvine and Mallory form a picturesque backdrop. The marginal campsites may be unattractive to backpackers—better sites can be found below, near Camp Lake.

 Camping

 Lake

 Wildflowers

⚐	**MILESTONES**	
▶1	0.0	Start at trailhead
▶2	3.5	Straight ahead at Grass Lake junction
▶3	4.5	Meysan Lake

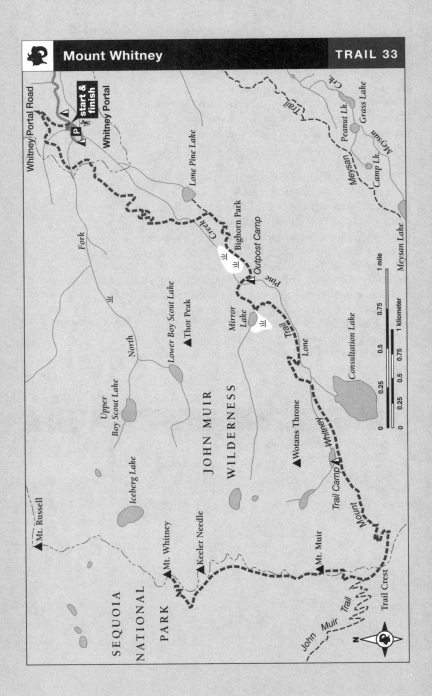

Whitney Portal Road

start & finish

Whitney Portal

Lone Pine Lake

Fork

North

Upper Boy Scout Lake

Lower Boy Scout Lake

Thor Peak

Iceberg Lake

Mt. Russell

SEQUOIA

NATIONAL

PARK

Mt. Whitney

Keeler Needle

JOHN MUIR

WILDERNESS

Mirror Lake

Bighorn Park

Outpost Camp

Consultation Lake

Wotans Throne

Trail Camp

Mt. Muir

Lone Pine Creek

Mount Whitney Trail

Trail Crest

John Muir Trail

McGee Cr.

Trail

Grass Lake

Peanut Lk.

Meysan

Camp Lk.

Meysan Lake

0   0.25   0.5   0.75   1 mile

0   0.25   0.5   0.75   1 kilometer

N

Mount Whitney

With a dramatic, towering, and vertical east face that cuts a familiar alpine profile as seen from the town of Lone Pine, more than 10,750 feet below, Mt. Whitney is one of North America's most impressive mountains. Not only is the view of the mountain quite exceptional, but the vista from the summit is equally impressive, a reward commensurate with the diligence required to reach the climax of the Sierra. To stand on top of the 14,494-foot summit is an extraordinary accomplishment.

While defined trail leads all the way to the summit, a Whitney climb is not necessarily a walk in the park. You must be in good physical condition to reach the summit and enjoy the journey along the way. Altitude is certainly a consideration, especially for those who reside at or near sea level. Spending a night in the campground at Whitney Portal prior to the start of a trip is a good way to begin the acclimatization process. Once on the trail, drink plenty of fluids, consume lots of high-energy foods, and continuously monitor your condition, as well as that of any companions. Slow your rate of ascent upon noticing any signs of mild altitude sickness. If symptoms persist, or worsen, make an immediate descent to lower altitudes. The proper equipment, including sunglasses, sunblock, plenty of food and water, and the appropriate clothing for the wide range of temperatures and weather conditions you might experience on this mountain, is also essential. Weather conditions run the gamut from intense sunlight and heat to sudden thunderstorms with torrential rains or hail. Snow can fall on Mt. Whitney during any month of the year!

TRAIL USE
Dayhike, Backpack, Run

LENGTH
22.0 miles, 11–15 hours

VERTICAL FEET
+7830/-1870/±19,400

DIFFICULTY
– 1 2 3 4 **5** +

TRAIL TYPE
Out & Back

FEATURES
Canyon
Mountain
Summit
Wildflowers
Great Views
Camping
Steep

FACILITIES
Campground
Picnic Area
Store
Cafe
Showers

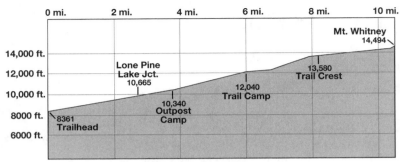

TRAIL 33 Mount Whitney Elevation Profile

Saying that Mt. Whitney is a coveted ascent is a huge understatement, as so many wish to climb the highest summit in the Lower 48 that the U.S. Forest Service long ago implemented a strict quota system to try to stem the tide from hordes of devotees attempting to reach the summit. Even with 100 dayhiker and 60 backpacker permits available per day ($15 per person), competition is so fierce that permits are granted by lottery (see page 190 for more information). In addition to the quota permit system, the Forest Service has also instituted a mandatory pack-out system within the Whitney Zone for removal of all human waste.

> **To stand on top of the 14,494-foot summit is an extraordinary accomplishment.**

The first question you need to answer before embarking on a Whitney climb is whether to do the ascent as a one-day hike or an overnight (or longer) backpack. The benefit of the one-day option is not having to carry a heavy backpack up the steep trail to basecamp. However, the 22-mile round trip demands that you be in top condition and get an early start for the long day ahead. Backpacking obviously requires you to carry more gear, but it allows you more time to acclimatize and to get up and down the mountain.

Best Time

Sunny and mild days between mid-July and mid-September are the ideal times for a climb of Mt. Whitney. Afternoon thunderstorms can occur at any time during that period and a hasty retreat should be undertaken during such conditions. Since so many desire to climb the highest peak in the continental U.S. and competition for permits is so fierce, many attempts occur outside of this window of usually fair and mild weather. Spring trips face the added obstacles of unstable weather and icy conditions, oftentimes requiring the use of ice axes and crampons. Autumn climbers must be fully prepared for sudden storms with the possibility of heavy snowfall and freezing temperatures.

Finding the Trail

From Lone Pine, head west from U.S. Highway 395 on the Whitney Portal Road and drive 13 miles to Whitney Portal, parking your vehicle either in the day-use or overnight parking lots. Whitney Portal Campground (fee, flush toilets, running water, bear boxes, and phone) and Whitney Trailhead Campground (walk-in, one-night limit, fee, flush toilets, running water, bear boxes, and phone) are close by. Whitney Portal also has a picnic area, restrooms, store, and cafe.

Logistics

All hikers in the Mt. Whitney Zone must obtain a wilderness dayhiking permit, and backpackers must obtain a permit for all overnight visits. Due to Mt. Whitney's popularity, hikers must enter a lottery at the beginning of the year or try for a walk-in permit. See page 190 for more details.

OPTIONS

Lone Pine Lake

Late-starting backpackers or dayhikers not up to the full-scale assault on Mt. Whitney can find a haven at lovely Lone Pine Lake. Turn left from the junction and head northeast about 200 yards to the east shore of the lake. Perched at the very edge of steep Lone Pine Creek canyon, the roughly oval lake is blessed with fine views down-canyon across the open, boulder-strewn shore. With no permanent inlet, the lake level is dependent on snowmelt from the previous winter's snowpack. Anglers can test their skill on a resident population of rainbow and brook trout, while campers can find spots to pitch their tents beneath foxtail pines above the southwest shore.

Trail Description

▶1 Your departure from **Whitney Portal** onto the **Mt. Whitney Trail** is heralded by an abundance of trailhead signs that may easily result in temporary sensory overload. Nearby is the receptacle for disposal of your waste pack-out kit upon the conclusion of your journey into the Whitney Zone. Away from this trailhead hoopla, the well-beaten path winds up the hillside through a mixed forest of red firs, Jeffrey pines, and mountain mahogany to the first switchback. Heading roughly east, cross chaparral-covered slopes with a fine view up the canyon of a falls on Lone Pine Creek. Cross an unnamed stream lined with lush vegetation and then follow a quarter-mile, ascending traverse to a boulder-hop of **North Fork Lone Pine Creek**. A steep mountaineer's route ascends this drainage to Iceberg Lake and technical routes on Whitney's east face. Farther up the trail, you cross the signed **John Muir Wilderness boundary**.

A mostly shadeless and steady climb ensues, incorporating numerous switchbacks on the climb up the canyon. If hot temperatures are forecast, try to avoid this 1.5-mile section of trail during the afternoon. Welcome relief comes in the form of a

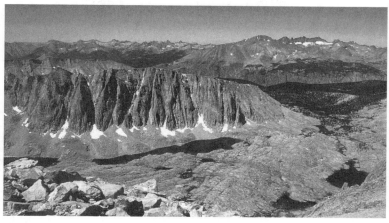

Western view *from summit of Mt. Whitney*

lodgepole-pine forest on the approach to a ford of Lone Pine Creek. Shortly beyond the ford is a junction ▶2 with the short spur trail to **Lone Pine Lake**.

Remaining on the Mt. Whitney Trail, you veer right at the Lone Pine Lake junction and gently stroll through a rocky wash beneath a light covering of pine into the Whitney Zone. Soon the stiff climb resumes on a series of switchbacks leading up and over a rocky slope to Bighorn Park, a large, willow-lined meadow sprinkled with colorful wildflowers. A gently graded path skirts the meadow to the south side and then turns north to a crossing of **Lone Pine Creek**. Just beyond the crossing, near a waterfall, is **Outpost Camp**, ▶3 with a number of slightly sloping, pine-shaded campsites.

Camping

Away from Outpost Camp, the trail immediately crosses **Mirror Creek** and ascends steep switchbacks alongside a wildflower-lined, tumbling stream. At the top of the climb, you boulder-hop back over the creek and pass through head-high willows to the southeast shore of **Mirror Lake**. ▶4 The lake is quite attractive, set in a deep cirque below

Wildflowers

Lake

the steep cliffs of Thor Peak. Anglers can test their skill on the brook trout rumored to live here, but campers will have to continue to Trail Camp, as camping has been banned here since 1972 due to severe overuse. Although camping is not allowed, the lovely surroundings of Mirror Lake make a fine rest or lunch stop.

More switchbacks lead out of Mirror Lake's basin on a stiff climb to the top of a ridge near timberline. Soon the rugged east wall of the Whitney massif appears over the top of Pinnacle Ridge. A more moderate climb leads across boulders and rocks, the rugged landscape broken intermittently by small pockets of soil with widely scattered wildflowers and tiny shrubs. A series of rock steps leads closer to **Lone Pine Creek**, as the trail eventually leads to a crossing of the creek on a rock bridge. Beyond the bridge, you continue to beautiful Trailside Meadows, where a colorful profusion of shooting stars, paintbrush, and columbine accents the deep green meadow grass lining the stream.

Wildflowers

Beyond this small oasis, you climb a nearly endless sea of rock, cross back over the creek, and continue to the vicinity of **Consultation Lake**, backdropped dramatically by Mt. Irvine and Mt. McAdie. Continue climbing steadily upward, weaving around boulders and over rock steps, before a stretch of gently graded trail heralds your approach

Camping

to **Trail Camp**. ►5 A short climb leads into the well-used camp.

Although the vast number and variety of campers may lend a circuslike atmosphere to **Trail Camp**, the setting, below the rugged east face of the High Sierra, is spectacular. To the north lies Wotan's Throne, with Pinnacle Ridge behind, while to the south, 13,680-foot Mt. McAdie and 13,770-foot Mt. Irvine form an amphitheater for the icy waters of Consultation Lake. Directly above the camp, 100 switchbacks lead to the low gap in the crest known as Trail Crest. This ever-present obstacle looms over prospective climbers hunkered down at Trail Camp, resulting in a restless night's sleep for many of them.

Leaving Trail Camp behind, increasingly steep trail leads to the bottom of the 100 switchbacks. Zigzag up the slope with ever expanding views to the east (Mt. Whitney becomes hidden behind

OPTIONS

Trail Camp

On just about any summer day, **Trail Camp** assumes the atmosphere of an expedition base camp. While multicolored tents flap in the breeze, expectant mountaineers sort their gear and check equipment, while others gaze at the route above, or check the skies for any hints at the weather. Still others wait trailside, querying returning summiteers about their experience higher up on the mountain. Not surprisingly, Trail Camp is not the place for isolationists in search of a solitary wilderness experience. Plenty of level campsites have been groomed by repeated use on the nearly barren soil surrounding the camp, but campers should not expect anything close to privacy.

With a maximum of 100 dayhikers and 60 backpackers departing from Whitney Portal each day, combined with an additional number of returnees and a handful of people finishing up their John Muir Trail thru-hikes, the potential exists for hundreds of people to pass through the camp on any given day. Some backpackers seek campsites in slightly less crowded areas away from the trail around Consultation Lake, but usually without much relief from the crush of visitors.

the Needles). About halfway up the slope, you climb across a shaded rock wall, where a seep may help create icy conditions; old iron railings add a wary sense of safety. The interminable switchbacks continue, as lingering snowfields may impede straightforward travel below the crest. Eventually, **Trail Crest** ▶6 is reached, where staggering views of the **Great Western Divide** appear to the west, encompassing a broad section of Sequoia National Park. Directly below, in a barren basin, lie the shimmering waters of Hitchcock Lakes. A short descent from Trail Crest leads to a junction with the **John Muir Trail**. ▶7

Great Views

Turn right and head north toward the summit of **Mt. Whitney** on a steady climb that follows the JMT along an airy ridge. The trail periodically dips into notches in the ridge that provide acrophobic vistas straight down the east face. Proceeding up the trail, you may notice the sunlight glinting off the metal roof of the **research hut** near the summit, built by the Smithsonian Institute in 1909. Approaching the final slope below the top, the grade increases and a variety of paths head toward the summit. Despite the number of routes, the way is obvious—head for the highest spot. Soon the roof of the hut appears over the horizon, and you stand atop the highest summit in the Lower 48. ▶8 The top of the peak is a broad, sloping plateau composed of jumbled slabs and boulders. Any adjective that attempts to capture the magnificence of the summit view seems inadequate. Suffice to say, it's a complete, 360-degree panorama, with each bearing of the compass offering something extraordinary to discover—a more than just reward for the toil necessary to reach this spectacular point. After fully enjoying the summit experience, retrace your steps back to **Whitney Portal**.

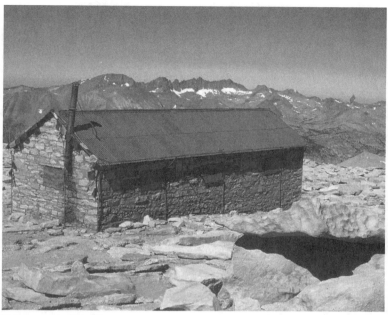

Hut *at summit of Mt. Whitney*

🚶	**MILESTONES**	
▶1	0.0	Start at Whitney Portal
▶2	2.75	Right at Lone Pine Lake junction
▶3	3.8	Outpost Camp
▶4	4.5	Mirror Lake
▶5	6.0	Trail Camp
▶6	8.2	Trail Crest
▶7	8.3	Right at John Muir Trail junction
▶8	11.0	Mt. Whitney

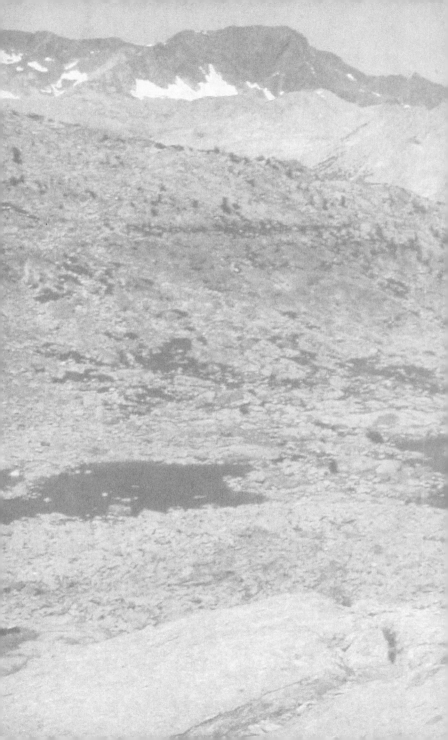

CHAPTER 4

John Muir Wilderness and East Kings Canyon

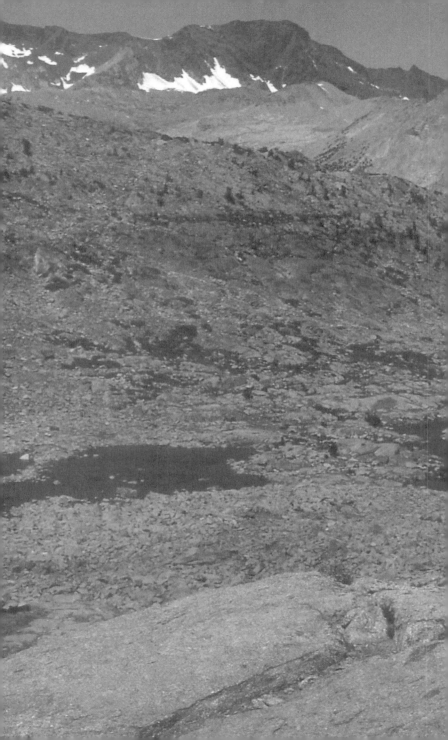

John Muir Wilderness and East Kings Canyon

Continuing the topography found to the south, this section of the eastern Sierra rises abruptly and dramatically from the plain of Owens Valley. Rugged mountains tower thousands of feet over the valley and the small communities dotting the plain. Trails in this area either dead-end at the base of impenetrable walls at the head of steep canyons, or they climb stiffly to high-elevation passes over the **Sierra Crest**. The magnificent beauty found in these mountains is well known to a host of recreationists, including hikers, backpackers, equestrians, alpinists, technical climbers, photographers, and anglers. Dramatic peaks, glacial-carved cirques, flower-bedecked meadows, shimmering alpine lakes, and deeply cleft canyons are all present in abundance, just waiting to be explored. Bounded by the Glacier Divide in the north and the main Sierra Crest to the east, the craggy terrain in this part of Kings Canyon National Park is the birthplace of two of the region's mightiest rivers, the **South Fork San Joaquin** and the **Middle Fork Kings**.

Highway 395 provides the principal access for trails in this area, with secondary roads heading west toward trailheads that eventually terminate in the shadow of the eastern Sierra. Similar to the region to the south described in Chapter 3, no roads cross the Sierra Crest and penetrate the remote backcountry of the park. The nearest trans-Sierra road, seasonally open Tioga Pass Road, is well to the north in Yosemite National Park. The trailheads provide jumping-off points for many multiday backpacks into some of the most remote wilderness in the Sierra. However, as the focus of this guide is limited to dayhikes and overnight backpacks, these adventures are not included within these pages.

All of the trails included in this chapter involve stiff climbs at high elevations. Trail users must be in good shape and well acclimated to experience the full enjoyment that these trips offer. Every one of the 17 trails described here travels to at least one beautiful alpine or subalpine lake, with many

Overleaf and opposite: *Palisade Basin*

trips visiting areas with several lakes and tarns. Midseason offers the added bonus of copious wildflowers gracing the meadows and lining the trails. No matter which trip is undertaken, the rugged spine of the High Sierra is magnificently omnipresent.

Trails 34–37 begin from trailheads in Onion Valley, with short climbs to **Robinson and Golden Trout lakes** and two longer adventures to the splendid terrain beyond **Kearsarge Pass**. Trails 38 and 39 are similar in that they both require long drives on rough dirt roads to reach remote trailheads and both climb steeply from near the edge of Owens Valley through exposed terrain. Trails 40 and 41 ascend canyons of **North Big Pine and South Big Pine creeks** to the stunning scenery beneath the **world-renowned Palisades**, an alpine mecca of 14,000-foot peaks and icy glaciers. The Bishop Pass Trail out of South Lake along South Fork Bishop Creek provides the access for Trips 42–45 to lakes on the east side of the crest, over **Bishop Pass** to lovely and verdant **Dusy Basin**, on the chapter's only semiloop (through the Chocolate Lakes) and a short hike to the **Treasure Lakes**. The next trip, Trail 46, is a half-day affair from South Lake Road that climbs shortly to a string of lakes known as **Tyee Lakes**. The next two trails begin at **Lake Sabrina**, with Trail 47 following Middle Fork Bishop Creek to lovely, lake-dotted Sabrina Basin and Trail 48 climbing to solitary **George Lake**. The final two trails head out from North Lake, with Trail 49 climbing stiffly but shortly to **Lamarck Lakes** and Trail 50 ascending over Piute Pass to the sweeping magnificence of lake-sprinkled and flower-covered **Humphreys Basin**.

Permits

Wilderness permits are required for all overnight stays in the backcountry of John Muir Wilderness and of Kings Canyon National Park. Trailhead quotas are in effect from May 1 to November 1 for eastside entry into John Muir Wilderness. Sixty percent of the daily quota is available by advanced reservation with a $5 per person fee. Reservations can be made up to six months before the start date of a trip by contacting the Wilderness Permit Office by phone (760-873-2483), or with a downloadable application (www.fs/fed. us/r5/inyo), reservations can also be submitted by fax (760-873-2484), or mail (Inyo National Forest, Wilderness Permit Office, 351 Pacu Lane, Bishop, CA 93514). The remaining 40 percent of the daily quota is available as walk-in permits. These free permits can be picked up beginning at 11 AM the day before the start of a trip through close of business the day of departure. All permits can be picked up at the Mono Basin Scenic Area

Visitors Center (Lee Vining), Mammoth Ranger Station (Mammoth Lakes), White Mountain Ranger Station (Bishop), or Eastern Sierra InterAgency Visitors Center (Lone Pine).

Maps

For John Muir Wilderness and East Kings Canyon, the USGS 7.5-minute (1:24,000 scale) topographic maps are listed below.

Trail 34: *Kearsarge Peak*
Trails 35–36: *Kearsarge Peak* and *Mt. Clarence King*
Trail 37: *Kearsarge Peak*
Trails 38–39: *Fish Springs* and *Split Mountain*
Trail 40: *Coyote Flat* and *Split Mountain*
Trail 41: *Coyote Flat, Split Mountain, Mt. Thompson,* and *North Palisade*
Trails 42–43: *Mt. Thompson* and *North Palisade*
Trails 44–46: *Mt. Thompson*
Trail 47: *Mt. Thompson* and *Mt. Darwin*
Trail 48: *Mt. Thompson*
Trail 49: *Mt. Darwin*
Trail 50: *Mt. Darwin, Mt. Tom, Mt. Hilgard,* and *Mt. Henry*

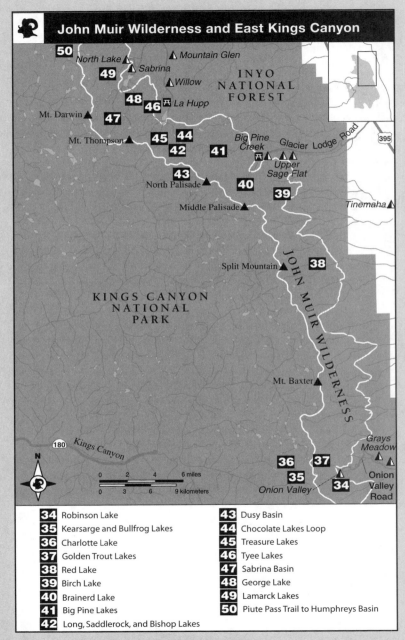

John Muir Wilderness and East Kings Canyon

INYO
NATIONAL
FOREST

North Lake
Mountain Glen
Sabrina
Willow
La Hupp
Mt. Darwin
Mt. Thompson
Big Pine Creek
Glacier Lodge Road
Upper Sage Flat
North Palisade
Middle Palisade
Tinemaha
395

Split Mountain

JOHN MUIR WILDERNESS

KINGS CANYON
NATIONAL
PARK

Mt. Baxter

Grays Meadow

Kings Canyon
180

Onion Valley Road

Onion Valley

N

0 2 4 6 miles
0 3 6 9 kilometers

34 Robinson Lake		**43** Dusy Basin	
35 Kearsarge and Bullfrog Lakes		**44** Chocolate Lakes Loop	
36 Charlotte Lake		**45** Treasure Lakes	
37 Golden Trout Lakes		**46** Tyee Lakes	
38 Red Lake		**47** Sabrina Basin	
39 Birch Lake		**48** George Lake	
40 Brainerd Lake		**49** Lamarck Lakes	
41 Big Pine Lakes		**50** Piute Pass Trail to Humphreys Basin	
42 Long, Saddlerock, and Bishop Lakes			

John Muir Wilderness and East Kings Canyon

TRAIL	Difficulty	Length	Type	USES & ACCESS	TERRAIN	FLORA & FAUNA	OTHER
34	3	3.0					
35	4	14.2					
36	4	16.5					
37	3	4.4					
38	5	9.0					
39	4	11.0					
40	4	10.0					
41	4	11.4					
42	3	8.6					
43	4	15.2					
44	3	7.2					
45	3	7.6					
46	3	6.5					
47	3	13.6					
48	3	6.6					
49	4	5.4					
50	4	14.4					

USES & ACCESS
- Dayhiking
- Backpacking
- Running
- Horses
- Dogs Allowed
- Child Friendly
- Handicapped Access

TYPE
- Loop
- Out & Back

DIFFICULTY
- 1 2 3 4 5 +
less   more

TERRAIN
- Canyon
- Mountain
- Summit
- Lake
- River or Stream
- Waterfall

FLORA & FAUNA
- Fall Colors
- Wildflowers
- Giant Sequoias

FEATURES
- Great Views
- Camping
- Swimming
- Secluded
- Steep
- Historic Interest
- Fishing

John Muir Wilderness and East Kings Canyon

Golden Trout Lakes 267

A short trail away from the usual hubbub found on the popular Kearsarge Pass Trail nearby leads to a trio of high lakes in the shadow of the eastern Sierra Crest. Along with the stunning terrain, the area offers anglers an opportunity to fish for the namesake trout.

TRAIL 37

Dayhike, Backpack,
Run, Horse,
Dogs Allowed
4.4 miles, Out & Back
Difficulty: 3

Red Lake 273

Solitude reigns supreme on this journey along a stiff dead-end trail to a remote eastern Sierra lake. The long drive on rough and dusty roads to the trailhead and the exposed climb to the lake seems to dissuade all but the most hardy of adventurers. Those who endure are rewarded with a beautiful lake in the shadow of the impressive east face of 14,058-foot Split Mountain, one of the 10 highest peaks in the range.

TRAIL 38

Dayhike, Backpack,
Run, Dogs Allowed
11.0 miles, Out & Back
Difficulty: 5

Birch Lake 279

Similar to Red Lake, the trip to Birch Lake requires a lengthy drive on dirt roads to the trailhead and a stiff climb from the edge of Owens Valley through shade-less terrain up a dead-end canyon to Birch Lake. The stunning east side scenery and lack of people will draw those who appreciate the road less traveled.

TRAIL 39

Dayhike, Backpack,
Run, Dogs Allowed
10.0 miles, Out & Back
Difficulty: 4

Brainerd Lake 283

The Palisades are well known to alpinists around the globe, and this trip into the Middle Palisades rivals any in the Sierra for sheer alpine beauty. At times the trail is both steep and poorly maintained but the awesome grandeur near Brainerd Lake more than compensates for these minor annoyances. Off-trail extensions to Finger Lake and Middle Palisade Glacier provide added bonuses.

TRAIL 40

Dayhike, Backpack,
Run, Horse,
Dogs Allowed
10.0 miles, Out & Back
Difficulty: 4

TRAIL 41

Dayhike, Backpack,
Run, Horse,
Dogs Allowed
11.4 miles, Semiloop
Difficulty: 4

Big Pine Lakes

The semiloop through the Big Pine Lakes is a quintessential High Sierra trip, visiting a bevy of gorgeous lakes beneath the towering summits of the Palisades. Side trails to additional lakes, as well as Sam Mack Meadow and the Palisade Glacier, offer so many wonderful diversions that one could easily spend an entire week in the upper North Fork Big Pine Creek basin.

TRAIL 42

Dayhike, Backpack,
Run, Horse,
Dogs Allowed
8.6 miles, Out & Back
Difficulty: 3

Long, Saddlerock, and Bishop Lakes

South Lake is the jumping-off point for many fine Sierra adventures, and this trip along the upper reaches of South Fork Bishop Creek is certainly no exception. The trail is popular, for good reason; travelers are treated to rushing streams, verdant meadows, colorful wildflowers, sparkling lakes, and towering peaks. The trail's popularity can make obtaining a wilderness permit challenging, with trailhead parking at a premium as well.

TRAIL 43

Dayhike, Backpack, Run
15.2 miles, Out & Back
Difficulty: 4

Dusy Basin

The verdant expanse of Dusy Basin is one of the most splendid alpine meadows in the Sierra. The basin is blessed with numerous lakes and tarns, rich meadows, a profusion of colorful wildflowers, refreshing little brooks, and a border of jagged alpine peaks. Don't forget the camera, since the dramatic scenery is some of the most photographed in the High Sierra.

Chocolate Lakes Loop......... 315

This relatively short semiloop leads around aptly named Chocolate Peak from the well-traveled Bishop Pass Trail to a string of picturesque lakes surrounded by outstanding scenery.

Dayhike, Backpack,
Run, Horse,
Dogs Allowed
7.2 miles, Semiloop
Difficulty: 3

Treasure Lakes............... 321

Excellent scenery and a variety of plant zones combine to make this short trip to the Treasure Lakes quite desirable. The upper lakes should offer a reasonable expectation of solitude as well.

Dayhike, Backpack, Run,
Horse, Dogs Allowed
7.6 miles, Out & Back
Difficulty: 3

Tyee Lakes.................... 327

Whether you're looking to fish, camp, swim, or just hike, the lightly used path to the high granite basin holding the Tyee Lakes fits the bill. Its short distance makes this trail well suited for a straightforward trip for recreationists of all ages.

Dayhike, Backpack,
Run, Horse,
Dogs Allowed
6.5 miles, Out & Back
Difficulty: 3

Sabrina Basin................. 333

The wonderfully picturesque Sabrina Basin near the headwaters of Middle Fork Bishop Creek holds a plethora of stunning lakes, which will leave day-trippers thirsty for more. There are numerous options for trip extensions to lakes off the beaten path via side trails and cross-country routes for those with more time. The scenery is magnificent, with towering peaks of the High Sierra rimming the basin.

Dayhike, Backpack, Run,
Horse, Dogs Allowed
13.6 miles, Out & Back
Difficulty: 3

TRAIL 48

Dayhike, Backpack,
Run, Horse,
Dogs Allowed
6.6 miles, Out & Back
Difficulty: 3

George Lake 341

A short climb away from the trail to Sabrina Basin
leads to lovely George Lake, a fine destination for a
quick dayhike or an easy overnight backpack. Despite
the short distance, the lake is lightly visited—mostly
by anglers on a quest for brook and rainbow trout.

TRAIL 49

Dayhike, Backpack,
Run, Horse,
Dogs Allowed
5.4 miles, Out & Back
Difficulty: 4

Lamarck Lakes 345

Two distinctly different lakes set in the shadow of
the eastern Sierra Crest provide worthy destinations
for a dayhike or overnight backpack. Although the
distance is minimal, the stiff climb may make the 2.7
miles to Upper Lamarck Lake seem a lot farther. The
nearby Wonder Lakes offer a fine trip extension for
cross-country enthusiasts.

TRAIL 50

Dayhike, Backpack,
Run, Horse,
Dogs Allowed
14.4 miles, Out & Back
Difficulty: 4

Piute Pass Trail
to Humphreys Basin 351

Surrounded by craggy peaks and ridges, Humphreys
Basin is one of the most picturesque spots in the
High Sierra, especially in midseason when the floor
of the basin is carpeted with colorful wildflowers.
The rigors of the stiff climb over Piute Pass are soon
forgotten amid the beauty of the sprawling basin,
sprinkled with lakes and bisected by delightful
brooks. Although most of the lakes are off-trail, the
open topography is easily negotiated by all but beginning recreationists.

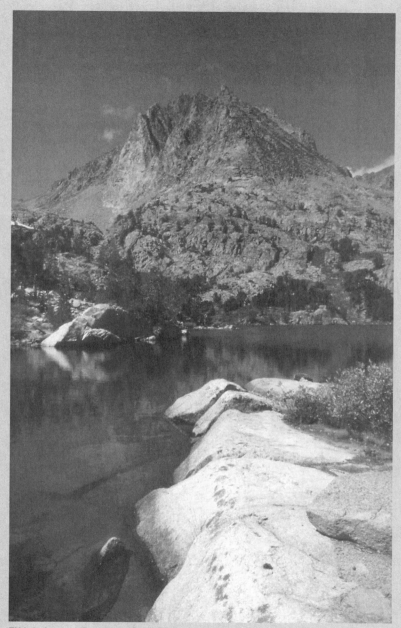

Fifth Lake and Two Eagle Peak *(Trail 41)*

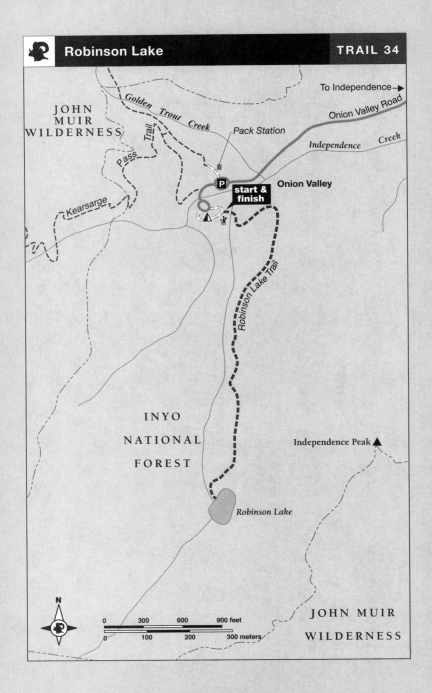

Robinson Lake TRAIL 34

To Independence →

JOHN
MUIR
WILDERNESS

Golden Trout Creek

Pack Station

Onion Valley Road

Independence Creek

Pass

Trail

P

Kearsarge

start & finish

Onion Valley

Robinson Lake Trail

INYO

NATIONAL

FOREST

Independence Peak ▲

Robinson Lake

N

| 0 | 300 | 600 | 900 feet |

| 0 | 100 | 200 | 300 meters |

JOHN MUIR

WILDERNESS

Robinson Lake

A short but sometimes steep hike leads to alpine splendor at Robinson Lake in the shadow of University and Independence peaks. Backpackers planning to overnight in the area, which is just outside the John Muir Wilderness, need not obtain a wilderness permit—a definite bonus for anyone who has been denied a permit for trails into the popular areas nearby.

Best Time

Snow blankets the area until mid-July following winters of average snowfall. The snow usually returns sometime in late October.

Finding the Trail

From the town of Independence, turn west from U.S. Highway 395 onto Market Street and head west following signs to Onion Valley. Drive 12.5 miles on the Onion Valley Road to the end and leave your vehicle in the expansive parking lot. Restrooms, running water, and a campground (fee, vault toilets, running water, and bear boxes) are available near the trailhead. Do not leave food or scented items in your car, as bears are active in Onion Valley.

Logistics

Backpackers must obtain a wilderness permit for all overnight visits. See page 238 for more details about how to obtain one.

TRAIL USE
Dayhike, Backpack, Run, Dogs Allowed

LENGTH
3.0 miles, 2 hours

VERTICAL FEET
+1325/±2650

DIFFICULTY
− 1 2 **3** 4 5 +

TRAIL TYPE
Out & Back

FEATURES
Mountain
Lake
Stream
Camping
Swimming
Steep

FACILITIES
Campground
Restrooms
Water
Stables

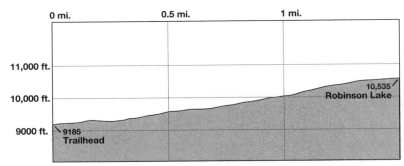

TRAIL 34 Robinson Lake Elevation Profile

Trail Description

Nestled in a steep,
horseshoe-shaped,
glacier-scoured
basin, sapphire-
blue Robinson Lake
emanates a bold,
alpine presence.

▶1 Follow directions given on a small sign near the parking area into the adjacent campground and continue along the access road to the start of the trail near Campsite 8. ▶2 From there, walk up a stone path, which doubles as a seasonal stream in early season, to sandy tread above and then switchback through aspens, whitebark pines, and foxtail pines on a moderately steep climb to a small, sloping basin sprinkled with scattered timber, site of some previous avalanches. Beyond the sloping basin, the grade eases to a more moderate ascent that leads near the west bank of Robinson Creek. Proceeding up the drainage, the grade increases again near a large patch of willows. Above the willows, you climb beside and then across a small stream, wind through a field of large boulders, and then crest the lip of the lake's basin. From there, a

Additional Challenges

From Robinson Lake, off-trail enthusiasts can follow a difficult, Class 2 cross-country route over University Pass into **Center Basin**, while mountaineers can follow a similarly rated route up 13,632-foot University Peak.

short stroll through an open area of rock, sand, and dwarf pines leads to the north shore of 10,535-foot **Robinson Lake**. ▶3

    Nestled in a steep, horseshoe-shaped, glacier-scoured basin, sapphire-blue Robinson Lake emanates a bold, alpine presence, with steep granite walls and talus slopes rising up from the lakeshore toward the summits of University and Independence peaks. Foxtail pines along the west shore shade a number of pleasant campsites. Rainbow and brook trout will tempt the angler.

≋ Lake

▲ Camping

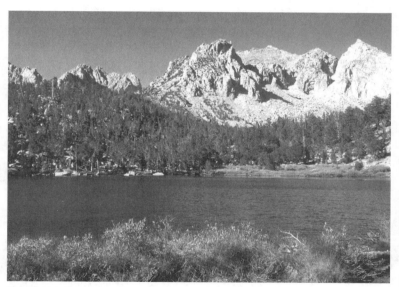

Robinson Lake

🚶	**MILESTONES**	
▶1	0.0	Start at parking area
▶2	0.1	Start of trail
▶3	1.5	Robinson Lake

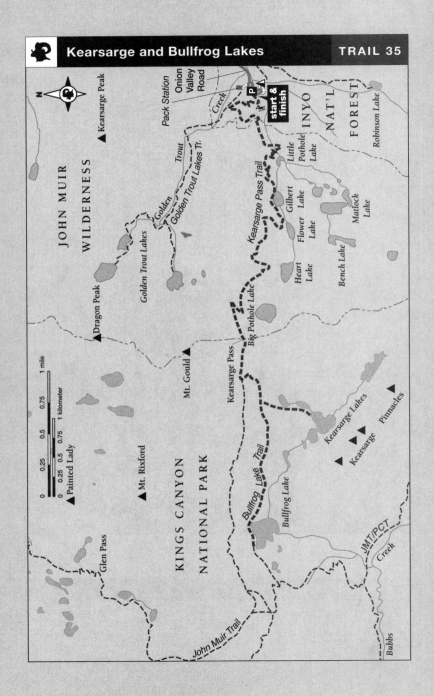

Kearsarge and Bullfrog Lakes

TRAIL 35

start & finish

Onion Valley Road

Pack Station

Kearsarge Peak

Creek

JOHN MUIR WILDERNESS

INYO NAT'L FOREST

Robinson Lake

Golden Trout

Golden Trout Lakes Tr.

Kearsarge Pass Trail

Little Pothole Lake

Gilbert Lake

Flower Lake

Matlock Lake

Golden Trout Lakes

Heart Lake

Bench Lake

Dragon Peak

Big Pothole Lake

Kearsarge Pass

Mt. Gould

1 mile

0.75

1 kilometer

0.5

0.25   0.5   0.75   1 kilometer

0   0.25   0.5   0.75

Painted Lady

Mt. Rixford

Bullfrog Lake Trail

Kearsarge Lakes

Kearsarge Pinnacles

Bullfrog Lake

KINGS CANYON NATIONAL PARK

Glen Pass

JMT/PCT

Creek

John Muir Trail

Bubbs

Kearsarge and Bullfrog Lakes

Kearsarge Pass provides one of the least difficult eastern gateways into the High Sierra. Consequently, the trail is heavily used, although getting to the pass still requires an elevation gain of over 2500 feet in 4.5 miles at high altitude. However, by Sierra standards, the climb is short and rarely at more than a moderate grade. Relative ease is not the only reason the Kearsarge Pass Trail is so popular with scores of hikers, backpackers, and equestrians, as the terrain is absolutely stunning. Serrated peaks, subalpine lakes, flower-filled meadows, rushing streams, and stunning views are the real draw in this portion of the Kings Canyon backcountry. With a string of five pretty lakes in the upper reaches of Independence Creek canyon, the real drama begins at the pass, where a sweeping view unfolds of Kearsarge and Bullfrog lakes backdropped by the row of rugged peaks known as the Kearsarge Pinnacles and, farther west, peaks of the Kings-Kern Divide across the deep chasm of Bubbs Creek. While the fine vista from Kearsarge Pass is a worthy goal for most day-trippers, the scenic lakes below are well worth a visit for strong hikers and backpackers.

Due to previously severe overuse, a one-night camping limit is in effect for Kearsarge Lakes and camping is banned outright at beautiful Bullfrog Lake. Bear canisters are required in the John Muir Wilderness east of Kearsarge Pass.

TRAIL USE
Dayhike, Backpack, Run, Horse
LENGTH
14.2 miles, 7–8 hours
VERTICAL FEET
+2700/-1450/±8300
DIFFICULTY
– 1 2 3 **4** 5 +
TRAIL TYPE
Out & Back

FEATURES
Mountain
Lake
Wildflowers
Great Views
Camping
Swimming
Fishing

FACILITIES
Campground
Restrooms
Water
Stables

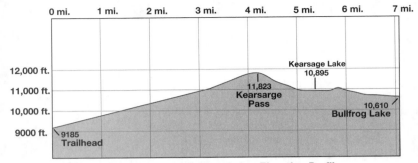

TRAIL 35 Kearsarge and Bullfrog Lakes Elevation Profile

Best Time

The pass is usually free of snow by mid-July. Wildflowers reach their peak from mid-July to early August.

Finding the Trail

From the town of Independence, turn west from U.S. Highway 395 onto Market Street and head west following signs to Onion Valley. Drive 12.5 miles on the Onion Valley Road to the end and leave your vehicle in the expansive parking lot. A campground (fee, vault toilets, running water, bear boxes), restrooms, and running water are available near the trailhead. Do not leave food or scented items in your car, as bears are active in Onion Valley.

Logistics

Backpackers must obtain a wilderness permit for all overnight visits. See page 238 for more details about how to obtain one.

Trail Description

▶1 The trail begins near the restrooms, climbing a sagebrush-covered hillside above to the first of many switchbacks to come. Nearing the drainage of Golden Trout Creek, you reach a junction with a short connector to the Golden Trout Lake Trail. ▶2 Remaining on the Kearsarge Pass Trail, proceed upslope through manzanita, mountain mahogany, and widely scattered red firs and limber pines toward the canyon of Independence Creek. Cross over the **John Muir Wilderness boundary** and continue to zigzag up the canyon, playing a game of hide and seek with the creek along the way. At one point during the climb, the stream is close enough for a thirst-slaking break. Continuing up the hillside, you have fine views down the canyon and across Owens Valley of the Inyo Mountains and south to the looming hulk of University Peak. A gently graded set of switchbacks leads to the first of the five lakes below Kearsarge Pass, **Little Pothole Lake**. ▶3 The willow-lined lake is attractively set **Lake** in a diminutive, half-moon-shaped basin, with waterfalls pouring down cliffs and flowing briefly through a patch of willows before entering the lake. A few overused campsites can be found around the shoreline beneath foxtail pines.

Additional switchbacks lead away from Little Pothole Lake and farther up the canyon. After a long talus slope, draw near to willow-lined Independence Creek again and soon reach **Gilbert Lake**. ▶4 Gilbert is an oval-shaped lake with a **Lake** pleasant-looking backdrop of craggy peaks. Grassy meadows dotted with clumps of willow provide straightforward access for anglers seeking to catch the resident brook and brown trout. However, the easy access and short distance from the trailhead means that the lake may be fished out by midseason. On the other hand, hot and dusty hikers will find the water well suited for an afternoon swim. As with Little Pothole Lake, a number of overused **Swimming** campsites ring the shoreline.

Lake

 Camping

The moderate, upward traverse culminates in a sweeping vista from 11,823-foot Kearsarge Pass, 6 with Kearsarge and Bullfrog lakes shimmering directly below.

The Kearsarge Pass Trail follows a gently graded course along the north side of Gilbert Lake before resuming the climb through a light pine forest along the creek. Soon you reach the vicinity of **Flower Lake**, ▶5 where a very short path heads down to the shoreline and a number of pleasant, pine-sheltered campsites. The lake hosts a population of brook trout but, similar to Gilbert Lake, the easy access limits the catch by midseason. If you wish to visit Heart Lake, head upstream cross-country from the west end of Flower Lake, as the Kearsarge Pass Trail climbs well away from this lake.

At the north end of Flower Lake, the switchbacks resume and the trail veers north and then east to attack the headwall of the canyon. Through scattered foxtail and whitebark pines, the trail zigzags up the headwall to an **overlook of Heart Lake**. More switchbacks lead through diminishing timber and rocky terrain to another overlook, this time of photogenic 11,256-foot Big Pothole Lake. Despite the sound of the name, given by Joseph N. LeConte, the lake is both deep and scenic, set in a horseshoe-shaped cirque beneath the very crest of the Sierra. A lack of vegetation lends an austere beauty to the lake's surroundings. A short cross-country ramble is necessary to reach the lake, where a few exposed campsites are scattered around the shore. Despite lacking a permanent inlet or outlet, the lake is reported to have a small population of brook trout.

Now the trail ascends stark, shalelike terrain via some long-legged switchbacks on the way toward the broad notch of **Kearsarge Pass**. A smattering of gnarled, dwarf whitebark pines defy the elements and cling desperately to the small pockets of soil, appearing more like wind-blasted shrubs than trees. The moderate, upward traverse culminates in a sweeping vista from 11,823-foot Kearsarge Pass, ▶6 with Kearsarge and Bullfrog lakes shimmering directly below. Above the lakes lie the rugged

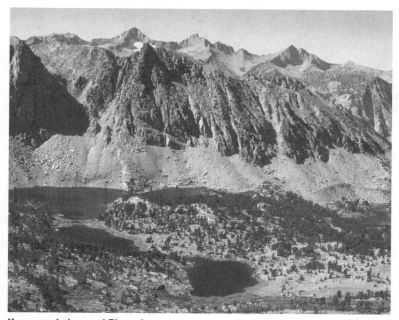

Kearsage Lakes and Pinnacles

Kearsarge Pinnacles, and farther west is the serrated crest of the Kings-Kern Divide. The high peak dominating the view to the west is 11,868-foot Mt. Bago. A number of signs greet you at the pass, welcoming you into Kings Canyon National Park.

A moderately steep descent from the pass leads high above the lake's basin and down toward more hospitable terrain. Near timberline is a junction with the Bullfrog Lake Trail. ►7

Turn left and follow the Bullfrog Lake Trail on a switchbacking descent that crosses several rivulets on the way toward the vicinity of **Kearsarge Lakes**. To reach the lakes, you'll have to head cross-country, as the U.S. Forest Service has long ago abandoned the maintenance of the laterals that used to provide trail access to the formerly overused lakes. At

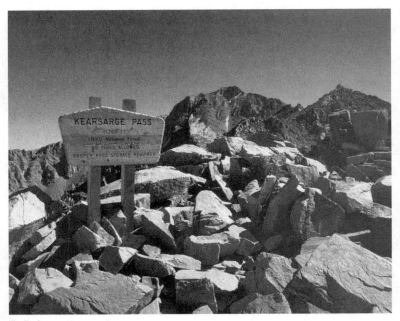

Trail sign *at Kearsage Pass*

0.25 mile from the junction, you may be able to find a faint use trail ▶8 that heads south across the granite basin through widely scattered clumps of whitebark pines to the lakes but, if not, the route-finding is straightforward. Passing by a couple of delightful tarns, you reach the largest lake (10,895 feet) ▶9 at 0.75 mile from the Bullfrog/Kearsarge junction. Tucked beneath the rugged wall of the **Kearsarge Pinnacles**, the lakes are quite pictur-esque. Backpackers are limited to a one-night stay at the lakes, and a couple of bear boxes are available for storing food and scented items. Anglers should find that the rainbow trout present a sufficient chal-lenge for testing their skills.

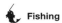 Camping

Fishing

To reach Bullfrog Lake, return to the **Bullfrog Lake Trail** ▶10 and head west through stunted pines and pockets of meadow on a moderate descent, hopping across numerous seasonal rivulets along the way. Soon the trail draws nearer to the main branch of the creek and proceeds through delightful open meadowlands on the way to Bullfrog Lake. Near the shore of this blue-green lake, ▶11 you soon realize why this area was such a popular camping destination, as the meadow-rimmed lake rivals any other in the Sierra for outstanding scenery. Across the deep trench of Bubbs Creek, the pyramidal summit of East Vidette rises sharply into the deep blue sky, providing a dramatic counterpoint to the usually placid waters of the lake. Above the shoreline, clumps of pine shelter former campsites graced with splendid views—nowadays fine spots for a picnic lunch.

🚶	**MILESTONES**	
▶1	0.0	Start at trailhead
▶2	0.3	Straight at junction
▶3	1.3	Little Pothole Lake
▶4	2.0	Gilbert Lake
▶5	2.25	Flower Lake
▶6	4.5	Kearsarge Pass
▶7	4.75	Left at Bullfrog Lake Trail junction
▶8	5.0	Left toward Kearsarge Lakes
▶9	5.5	Kearsarge Lake
▶10	6.0	Left on Bullfrog Lake Trail
▶11	7.1	Bullfrog Lake

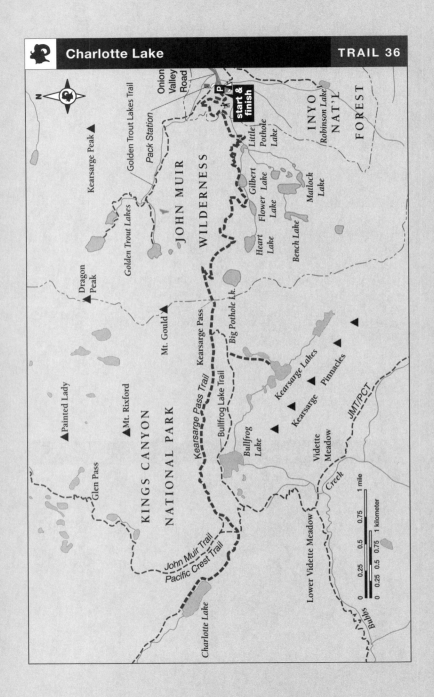

N

Onion
Valley
Road

start &
finish

P

Golden Trout Lakes Trail

Pack Station

Kearsarge Peak ▲

Little
Pothole
Lake

J O H N M U I R

W I L D E R N E S S

Gilbert
Lake

Flower
Lake

Heart
Lake

Bench Lake

Matlock
Lake

I N Y O

Robinson Lake

N A T ' L

F O R E S T

Golden Trout Lakes

Dragon
Peak ▲

Mt. Gould ▲

Kearsarge Pass

Big Pothole Lk.

Kearsarge Pass Trail

Bullfrog Lake Trail

Painted Lady ▲

▲Mt. Rixford

K I N G S C A N Y O N

N A T I O N A L P A R K

Glen Pass

Kearsarge Lakes

Kearsarge

Pinnacles

JMT/PCT

Bullfrog
Lake

Vidette
Meadow

Creek

John Muir Trail

Pacific Crest Trail

Lower Vidette Meadow

Bubbs

Charlotte Lake

1 mile

1 kilometer

0.75

0.5

0.25

0

0.75

0.5

0.25

0

Charlotte Lake

The 16.5-mile round-trip distance means that the trip over Kearsarge Pass to Charlotte Lake is better suited for backpackers, although strong hikers without a heavy backpack can get there and back in a long day. The rewards are numerous, with splendid scenery along the entire route, including the five lakes in upper Independence Creek canyon, sweeping views from Kearsarge Pass and vicinity, and the picturesque terrain around Charlotte Lake. Backpackers should be aware that the Park Service has limited camping to one night at Charlotte Lake.

Best Time

The pass is usually free of snow by mid-July. Wildflowers reach their peak from mid-July to early August.

Finding the Trail

From the town of Independence, turn west from U.S. Highway 395 onto Market Street and head west following signs to Onion Valley. Drive 12.5 miles on the Onion Valley Road to the end and leave your vehicle in the expansive parking lot. Restrooms, running water, and a campground (fee, vault toilets, running water, and bear boxes) are available near the trailhead. Do not leave food or scented items in your car, as bears are active in Onion Valley.

Logistics

Backpackers must obtain a wilderness permit for all overnight visits. See page 238 for more details about how to obtain one.

TRAIL USE
Dayhike, Backpack, Run, Horse

LENGTH
16.5 miles, 8–9 hours

VERTICAL FEET
+2700/-1450/±8300

DIFFICULTY
– 1 2 3 **4** 5 +

TRAIL TYPE
Out & Back

FEATURES
Mountain
Lake
Wildflowers
Great Views
Camping
Swimming
Fishing

FACILITIES
Campground
Restrooms
Water
Stables

261

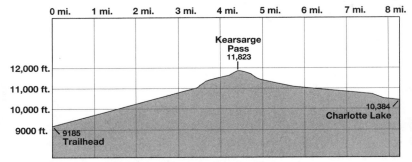

TRAIL 36　Charlotte Lake Elevation Profile

Trail Description

▶1 The trail begins near the restrooms, climbing a sagebrush-covered hillside above to the first of many switchbacks to come. Nearing the drainage of Golden Trout Creek, you reach a junction with a short connector to the Golden Trout Lake Trail. ▶2 Remaining on the Kearsarge Pass Trail, proceed upslope through manzanita, mountain mahogany, and widely scattered red firs and limber pines toward the canyon of Independence Creek. Cross over the **John Muir Wilderness boundary** and continue to zigzag up the canyon, playing a game of hide and seek with the creek along the way. At one point during the climb, the stream is close enough for a thirst-slaking break. Continuing up the hillside, you have fine views down-canyon and across Owens Valley of the Inyo Mountains and south to the looming hulk of University Peak. A gently graded set of switchbacks leads to the first of the five lakes below Kearsarge Pass, **Little Pothole Lake**. ▶3 The willow-lined lake is attractively set in a diminutive, half-moon-shaped basin, with waterfalls pouring down cliffs and flowing briefly through a patch of willows before entering the lake. A few overused campsites can be found around the shoreline beneath foxtail pines.

Lake

Additional switchbacks lead away from Little Pothole Lake and farther up-canyon. After a long talus slope, draw near to the willow-lined Independence Creek again and soon reach **Gilbert Lake**. ►4 Gilbert is an oval-shaped lake with a **Lake** pleasant-looking backdrop of craggy peaks. Grassy meadows dotted with clumps of willow provide straightforward access for anglers seeking to catch the resident brook and brown trout. However, the easy access and short distance from the trailhead means that the lake may be fished out by midseason. On the other hand, hot and dusty hikers will find the water well suited for an afternoon swim. As with Little Pothole Lake, a number of overused campsites **Swimming** ring the shoreline.

The Kearsarge Pass Trail follows a gently graded course along the north side of Gilbert Lake before resuming the climb through a light pine forest along the creek. Soon you reach the vicinity of **Flower Lake**, ►5 where a very short path heads down to the shoreline and a number of pleasant, pine-sheltered campsites. The lake hosts a population of brook **▲ Camping** trout but, similar to Gilbert Lake, the easy access limits the catch by midseason. If you wish to visit Heart Lake, head upstream cross-country from the west end of Flower Lake, as the Kearsarge Pass Trail climbs well away from the lake.

At the north end of Flower Lake, the switchbacks resume and the trail veers north and then east to attack the headwall of the canyon. Through scattered foxtail and whitebark pines, the trail zigzags up the headwall to an **overlook of Heart Lake**. More switchbacks lead through diminishing timber and rocky terrain to another overlook, this time of photogenic 11,256-foot Big Pothole Lake. Despite the sound of the name, given by Joseph N. LeConte, the lake is both deep and scenic, set in a horseshoe-shaped cirque beneath the very crest of the Sierra. A lack of vegetation lends an austere beauty to the lake's surroundings. A short cross-country ramble is necessary to reach the lake, where a few exposed campsites are scattered around the shore. Despite lacking a permanent inlet or outlet, the lake is reported to have a small population of brook trout.

Now the trail ascends stark, shalelike terrain via some long-legged switchbacks on the way toward the broad notch of Kearsarge Pass. A smattering of gnarled, dwarf whitebark pines defy the elements and cling desperately to the small pockets of soil, appearing more like wind-blasted shrubs than trees. The moderate, upward traverse culminates in a sweeping vista from 11,823-foot **Kearsarge Pass**, ▶6 with Kearsarge and Bullfrog lakes shimmering directly below. Above the lakes lie the rugged Kearsarge Pinnacles and farther west is the serrated crest of the Kings-Kern Divide. The high peak dominating the view to the west is 11,868-foot Mt. Bago. A number of signs greet you at the pass, welcoming you into Kings Canyon National Park.

A moderately steep descent from the pass leads high above the lake's basin and down toward more hospitable terrain. Near timberline is a junction with the Bullfrog Lake Trail. ▶7 Remain on the Kearsarge Pass Trail, as meadow grass, clumps of willow, and seasonal rivulets soften the otherwise rocky slopes. Fine views of Kearsarge Lakes and Kearsarge Pinnacles are constant companions along the moderate descent and, farther down the trail, **Bullfrog Lake** makes a stunning appearance, framed by the spiked summits of East Vidette and West Vidette across the deep chasm of Bubbs Creek. Junction and Center peaks further enhance the fine vista to the south. Eventually the expansive view is diminished a little by a scattered to light forest of whitebark and foxtail pines. Proceed to a Y-junction ▶8 with a connector to the **John Muir Trail** that provides a shortcut to Rae Lakes. Veer left, remaining on the Kearsarge Pass Trail, and head south and

> At the northwest end, a splayed, V-shaped cleft allows the waters from the lake to tumble down the canyon of Charlotte Creek and late in the day lets in a rosy glow from dramatic sunsets.

then southwest breaking out of the trees to cross a large, sandy flat on the way to a four-way junction ▶9 with the JMT and Charlotte Lake Trail.

From the junction, head west and then north-west on a winding descent through forest to the east shore of 10,384-foot **Charlotte Lake**. ▶10 The delightful lake is rimmed by scattered pines and nearly surrounded by high hills. At the northwest end, a splayed, V-shaped cleft allows the waters from the lake to tumble down the canyon of Charlotte Creek and late in the day lets in a rosy glow from dramatic sunsets. As the only lake with decent campsites easily accessible from the JMT between Forester and Glen passes, the lake does receive a fair share of thru-hikers. Nonetheless, sufficient campsites are spread around the shoreline, with bear boxes on the north side of the lake. The Park Service also has a ranger cabin near the north shore's midpoint. Anglers will be tempted by fair-size rainbow and brook trout.

 Lake

 Camping

 Fishing

🚶	**MILESTONES**	
▶1	0.0	Start at trailhead
▶2	0.3	Straight at junction
▶3	1.3	Little Pothole Lake
▶4	2.0	Gilbert Lake
▶5	2.25	Flower Lake
▶6	4.5	Kearsarge Pass
▶7	4.75	Straight at Bullfrog Lake Trail junction
▶8	7.2	Left at junction
▶9	7.5	Straight at Charlotte Lake junction
▶10	8.25	Charlotte Lake

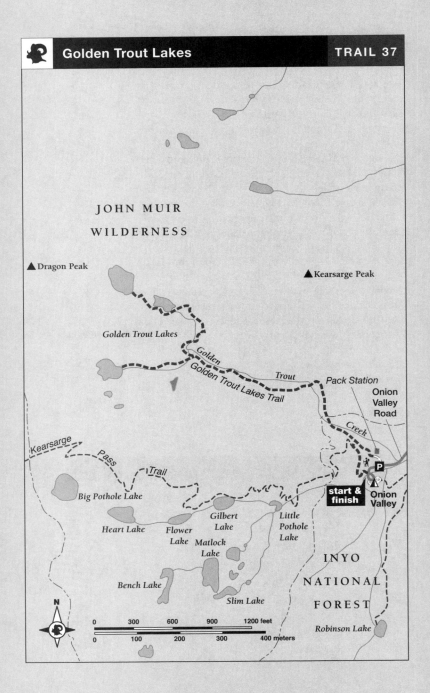

JOHN MUIR

WILDERNESS

▲ Dragon Peak   ▲ Kearsarge Peak

Golden Trout Lakes

Golden

Trout   *Pack Station*

Golden Trout Lakes Trail   Onion
                                      Valley
                                      Road

Creek

Kearsarge

Pass

Trail

**start &
finish**   Onion Valley

Big Pothole Lake

                              Little
Heart Lake   Gilbert   Pothole
        Flower   Lake   Lake   INYO
         Lake   Matlock
                 Lake   NATIONAL

Bench Lake   FOREST
              Slim Lake

N

0   300   600   900   1200 feet
0   100   200   300   400 meters   *Robinson Lake*

Golden Trout Lakes

The three lakes generally referred to as the Golden Trout Lakes (only the southernmost lake has the official name) provide fine destinations for either a pleasant dayhike or an overnight backpack. The lakes are cradled in talus-filled cirques just below the Sierra Crest in the shadow of Mt. Gould and Dragon Peak. Very few trails allow hikers into such an austere alpine environment with so little effort. Although the Kearsarge Pass Trail in the next canyon south is one of the most popular eastside trails in the High Sierra, relatively few hikers find their way up the unmaintained Golden Trout Lakes Trail. The trail is not in the best of shape but, despite the condition, the route to the lakes is straightforward and the extraordinary scenery more than makes up for a few indistinct sections.

Best Time

Most of the trail is generally snow-free by early July, but the east-facing cirques that hold the lakes may cling to snow until mid-month. Wildflowers are best from mid-July to early August.

Finding the Trail

From the town of Independence, turn west from U.S. Highway 395 onto Market Street and head west following signs to Onion Valley. Drive 12.5 miles on the Onion Valley Road to the end and leave your vehicle in the expansive parking lot. Restrooms, running water, and a campground (fee, vault toilets, running water, and bear boxes) are available near

TRAIL USE
Dayhike, Backpack,
Run, Horse,
Dogs Allowed
LENGTH
4.4 miles, 2–3 hours
VERTICAL FEET
+2300/-100/±4800
DIFFICULTY
– 1 2 **3** 4 5 +
TRAIL TYPE
Out & Back

FEATURES
Mountain
Lake
Wildflowers
Camping
Swimming
Fishing

FACILITIES
Campground
Restrooms
Water
Stables

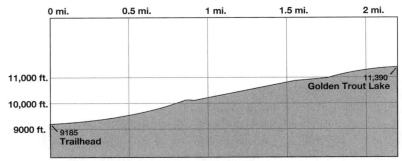

| 0 mi. | 0.5 mi. | 1 mi. | 1.5 mi. | 2 mi. |

11,000 ft.

11,390
Golden Trout Lake

10,000 ft.

9000 ft.

9185
Trailhead

TRAIL 37   Golden Trout Lakes Elevation Profile

the trailhead. Do not leave food or scented items in your car, as bears are active in Onion Valley.

Logistics

Backpackers must obtain a wilderness permit for all overnight visits. See page 238 for more details about how to obtain one.

Trail Description

▶1 The trail begins near the restrooms, climbing a sagebrush-covered hillside above to a switchback. Nearing the drainage of Golden Trout Creek, you reach a junction with a short connector to the **Golden Trout Lake Trail**. ▶2

Leave the Kearsarge Pass Trail and drop shortly to a junction ▶3 with a trail from the pack station and then head upstream along **Golden Trout Creek** through open pinyon pine and sagebrush terrain. Views up-canyon include Golden Trout Fall. Riparian vegetation appears where the trail closely follows a stretch of the creek, crosses the creek, and immediately enters the John Muir Wilderness.

Continue up the canyon on a winding climb through loose rock that leads above the waterfall. From there, pass through a flower-filled gully and

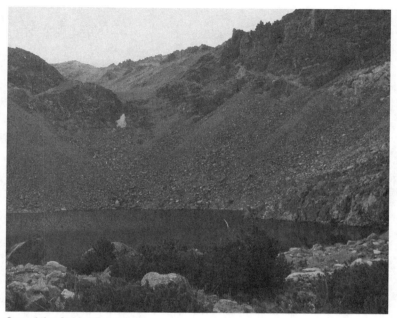

One of the Golden Trout Lakes

cross back over Golden Trout Creek. Beyond the second creek crossing, the tread becomes faint and a little hard to follow in places, especially in areas filled with talus and boulders. However, the route is obvious—head upstream through the narrow canyon. The trail makes two close fords of the creek, but the tread is so faint here that these crossings are easily missed. Eventually, you climb less steep terrain on the way to a lush meadow near where the creek forks into two branches. Passable campsites are nearby on a low rise. ▶4

To reach Golden Trout Lake, the southernmost lake bearing the official name, cross the left-hand branch of the creek and head west along the north bank through gnarled whitebark pines and a few foxtail pines. Once again, the tread is a bit sketchy, but the route is obvious. Continue up the creek to

 Wildflowers

 Camping

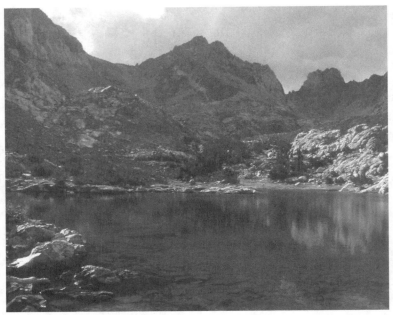

One of the Golden Trout Lakes

 Lake

 Camping

Fishing

the east shore of **Golden Trout Lake**, ▶5 where a few matted shrubs and some widely scattered dwarf whitebark pines vainly attempt to soften the boulder- and talus-filled, glacier-carved amphitheater. The apex of this rugged amphitheater is 13,005-foot **Mt. Gould**. A pair of fine campsites near the outlet may tempt backpackers, while anglers can test their skill on brook trout and the lake's namesake fish. Experienced off-trail enthusiasts can continue up-canyon, scrambling over boulders to **Dragon Pass**, a 12,800-foot notch halfway between Mt. Gould and Dragon Peak.

Unnamed Lakes

The USGS 7.5-minute map shows a trail that follows the right-hand branch of **Golden Trout Creek** to a pair of unnamed tarns east of **Dragon Peak**. Although this path has mostly disappeared over time, the route is an easily managed cross-country trek. From where the creek forks, follow the right-hand branch around a meadow, over the creek, and up the canyon to the lower lake. From there, the route to the upper lake is just as straightforward. Both tarns are quite scenic, picturesquely backdropped by the multihued flanks of Dragon Peak. A few campsites can be found at both lakes.

MILESTONES

►1	0.0	Start at Onion Valley Trailhead
►2	0.3	Right at junction of connector
►3	0.35	Left at junction of Golden Trout Lakes Trail
►4	1.7	Left at fork of Golden Trout Creek
►5	2.2	Golden Trout Lake

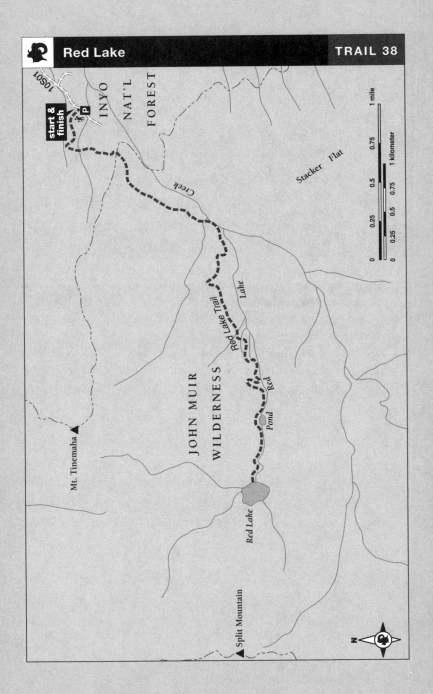

Red Lake

If there existed a list for lonely spots in the eastern High Sierra within a day's walk of a trailhead, then the 4.5-mile trip to Red Lake would surely be included. Of course, Red Lake would be included because of the long, dusty drive on dirt roads necessary to reach the trailhead and the trail's steep and sweltering climb. So, why bother with such a trip? The rewards for such an arduous journey are solitude and scenery. So few hikers make the trip to Red Lake that trailhead quotas weren't even implemented until 2002, when all trails in the Inyo National Forest received a quota, whether they needed one or not. The few who do make the trip will experience a superbly picturesque lake backdropped by the impressive east face of 14,058-foot Split Mountain, culminating in twin summits separated by a narrow cleft.

Before setting out on a journey to Red Lake, make sure your vehicle is roadworthy. In addition, get an early start to avoid making the climb during the hot part of the day. Also, be sure to pack along plenty of extra water. With these precautions, your visit to one of the eastern Sierra's most remote and scenic areas has the potential to be quite pleasant despite the rugged conditions.

TRAIL USE
Dayhike, Backpack,
Run, Dogs Allowed

LENGTH
9.0 miles, 5 hours

VERTICAL FEET
+4200/-275/±8950

DIFFICULTY
– 1 2 3 4 **5** +

TRAIL TYPE
Out & Back

FEATURES
Mountain
Lake
Wildflowers
Camping
Swimming
Secluded
Steep
Fishing

FACILITIES
None

Best Time

Lying somewhat in the rain shadow of the Sierra, the terrain around Red Lake tends to shed snow a little earlier than areas closer to the crest. Snow-free conditions usually begin in late June and continue through October in most years.

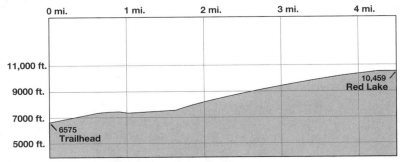

TRAIL 38 Red Lake Elevation Profile

Finding the Trail

In some ways, getting to the trailhead may present just as great a challenge as the hike to the lake. A 12-mile section of dirt road should be considered part of the adventure—plan on an hour-long drive from Big Pine to the trailhead. In the center of Big Pine, turn west from U.S. Highway 395 onto Crocker Road, which soon becomes Glacier Lodge Road outside of town, and proceed 2.75 miles to McMurry Meadows Road (FSR 9S03). Turn left onto a dirt road and immediately bear left, bypassing a 4WD road on the right. After a very brief climb, veer right, pass below a power line, and continue on McMurry Meadows Road, ignoring lesser roads along the way. Pass the road to the Birch Lake trailhead at 5.75 miles from Glacier Lodge Road, cross Birch Creek, proceed past McMurry Meadows to a Y-junction at 7 miles and bear left. Immediately past the junction, a small, crude sign marked RED LAKE TRAIL may provide some reassurance that you're still on the right road.

A quarter-mile descent leads across Fuller Creek to a T-junction just beyond. Here, turn left, parallel the creek downstream on rough road, cross back over the creek to the north side, and continue downstream to a major intersection, 9 miles from Glacier Lodge Road, where a locked gate bars forward progress. Turn right at the intersection and head south for ¾ mile, crossing Fuller and Tinemaha creeks on the way to a T-junction. Turn right (west) and follow FS 10S01 another 2 miles to a fork. A small sign nearby directs you to veer left for the trailhead parking area and right to the start of the trail. The nearest campgrounds are up the Glacier Lodge Road outside of the town of Big Pine.

Logistics

Backpackers must obtain a wilderness permit for all overnight visits. See page 238 for more details about how to obtain one.

Trail Description

▶1 Follow the north branch of the road uphill toward the start of single-track trail near a water diversion structure. Although the south branch of the road heads more directly toward Red Mountain Creek, the trail does not continue up the steep, brush-choked canyon. Climb moderately steeply up the hillside, paralleling a spring-fed tributary of the creek. Soon the trail bends south, crosses a seasonal drainage, and continues across a sagebrush-covered hillside. Without the customary fanfare from a sign, you enter the **John Muir Wilderness** and follow a curving ascent into **Red Mountain Creek canyon**, where the trail assumes a more gently ascending grade. The trail draws near to the creek for a brief stretch, before a steep, zigzagging ascent leads away from the creek, up a gully, and across a seasonal stream toward some steep cliffs. Cross a rocky wash and zigzag up the hillside to a thicket of vegetation, where a cool and refreshing stream courses down a cleft of rock. A few lonely pines put in an appearance, lending hope that all this climbing

Surrounded by pockets of willow and widely scattered whitebark pines, Red Lake sits dramatically below the steep talus slope and vertical walls of 14,058-foot Split Mountain.

 Steep

will eventually lead to more mountainlike terrain above.

Soon cross another lushly lined stream, step over a rocky wash, and emerge onto the slope above **Red Mountain Creek** once more. As you near the willow-lined stream, a switchback leads away on a lengthy diagonal ascent across a hillside, with improving views of the Inyo Mountains across Owens Valley. Another switchback leads back to the canyon and a fine view to the west of Split Mountain. After some more climbing, the grade gratefully levels off on the approach to an unnamed pond. ▶2 The view of **Split Mountain** across the surface of this pond is quite impressive. A few decent campsites on the far shoreline will surely tempt overnighters after the stiff and exposed climb.

The trail passes halfway around the north shore of the pond before petering out in a pile of talus, and then reappearing briefly beyond the pond (additional campsites) before disappearing for good beneath a talus slide. A quarter-mile scramble from there leads to the east shore of 10,459-foot **Red Lake**. ▶3 Surrounded by pockets of willow and widely scattered whitebark pines, Red Lake sits dramatically below the steep talus slope and vertical walls of 14,058-foot Split Mountain. Crude campsites suggest that the camping may be better back along the creek or near the unnamed pond. Anglers may wish to ply the waters of the lake in search of golden trout.

 Great Views

 Camping

 Lake

Fishing

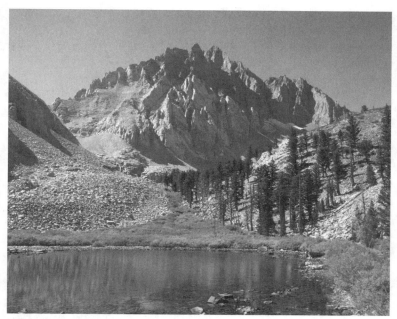

Pond and Split Mountain *from Red Lake Trail*

MILESTONES

▶1 0.0 Start at parking area
▶2 3.75 Unnamed pond
▶3 4.5 Red Lake

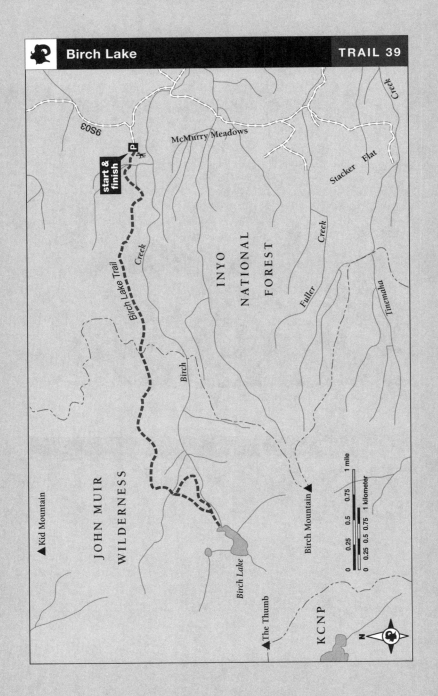

9S03

McMurry Meadows

start & finish

P

Birch Lake Trail

Creek

INYO   NATIONAL   FOREST

Stacker Flat

Creek

Fuller

Creek

Tinemaha

Birch

JOHN MUIR

WILDERNESS

▲ Kid Mountain

Birch Mountain ▲

Birch Lake

▲ The Thumb

KCNP

N

0   0.25   0.5   0.75   1 kilometer
0   0.25   0.5   0.75   1 mile

Birch Lake

Access via dirt road combined with a low-elevation trailhead on the east edge of Owens Valley and an infrequently maintained trail dissuade many hikers from contemplating a trip into the dead-end canyon of Birch Creek to Birch Lake. Despite these perceived drawbacks, the lake is quite scenic, reposing in the broad canyon of aspen-lined Birch Creek between the summits of the Thumb and Birch Mountain.

Best Time

Late June through mid-October is the snow-free season in this area on the east side of the Sierra Crest.

Finding the Trail

In the center of Big Pine, turn west from U.S. Highway 395 onto Crocker Road, which soon becomes Glacier Lodge Road outside of town, and proceed 2.75 miles to McMurry Meadows Road (FSR 9S03). Turn left onto the dirt road and immediately bear left, bypassing a 4WD road on the right. After a very brief climb, veer right, pass below a power line, and continue on McMurry Meadows Road, ignoring lesser roads along the way. Reach a junction with the road to the Birch Lake trailhead at 5.75 miles from Glacier Lodge Road and turn right (north) just before Birch Creek. Continue up the less traveled roadbed for 0.6 mile to a T-junction. Here, bear right and drive another 0.1 mile to a small parking area near a closed gate. The nearest

TRAIL USE
Dayhike, Backpack, Run, Dogs Allowed

LENGTH
11.0 miles, 5–6 hours

VERTICAL FEET
+4625/-300/±9850

DIFFICULTY
− 1 2 3 **4** 5 +

TRAIL TYPE
Out & Back

FEATURES
Mountain
Lake
Wildflowers
Camping
Swimming
Secluded
Fishing

FACILITIES
None

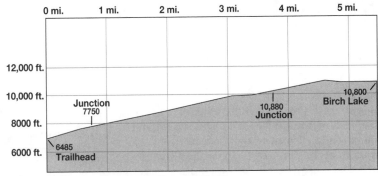

TRAIL 39 Birch Lake Elevation Profile

campgrounds are up the Glacier Lodge Road outside of the town of Big Pine.

Logistics

Backpackers must obtain a wilderness permit for all overnight visits. See page 238 for more details about how to obtain one.

Trail Description

Wildflowers

▶1 Initially, the route follows the closed 4WD road past the gate and about 100 yards to a trailhead sign. Continue up the road through a field of tall grass and occasional patches of wild rose, followed by alternating sections of sagebrush scrub and meadows on the way to a Y-junction. ▶2 Although you may feel inclined to follow the left-hand road toward Birch Creek, the actual route follows the right-hand branch along a seasonal drainage. Eventually the road narrows to single-track trail that heads up a sandy wash. A switchback leads out of the wash and onto more solid footing, with fine views to the east of **Owens Lake and the White Mountains**. A steady, winding climb proceeds over a hill and into a canyon of a seasonal tributary of **Birch Creek**. Climb moderately steeply up this tributary, past a tiny, spring-fed stream and out of the drainage to an unsigned junction on a grassy slope. ▶3

Bear left at the junction and follow the horse-shoe curve of the trail around a side canyon and then up to the top of a rise with a spectacular view of **Owens Valley**. From there, drop off the rise and descend into the next drainage, where the tread becomes a bit sketchy, splitting into two paths, each offering a slightly different approach to **Birch Lake**. The route as shown on the USGS 7.5-minute map continues up the drainage, crosses the creek above a spring, and then heads south on a three-quarter-mile traverse into Birch Creek canyon just below the lake. The other path immediately crosses the drainage and heads straight into Birch Creek canyon well below the lake. Whichever of the two paths you elect to follow, once you reach Birch Creek canyon, the scenery is quite dramatic. A number of primitive campsites can be found along the tumbling creek below the lake, which is reached by proceeding upstream through open terrain and over talus to a pretty meadow just below the lake. A short distance above the meadow is **Birch Lake**, ▶4 lying in a broad valley with excellent views up-canyon of the **Sierra Crest**. The lake offers a fine opportunity for anglers to test their skill on the resident cutthroat trout.

 Camping

 Lake

![hiker]	MILESTONES		
▶1	0.0	Start at parking area	
▶2	0.75	Right at Y-junction	
▶3	3.75	Left at junction	
▶4	5.5	Birch Lake	

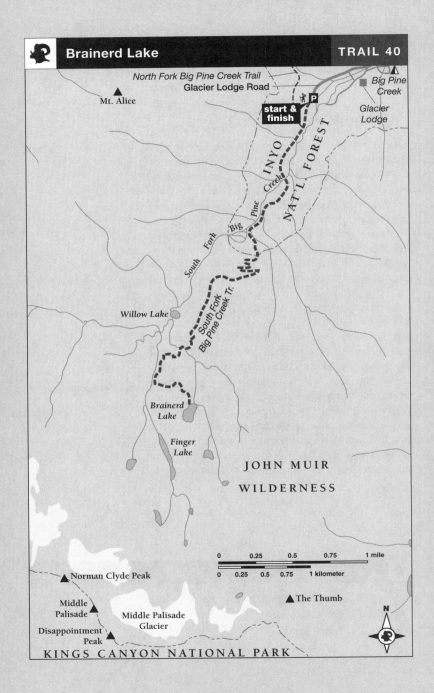

Brainerd Lake

TRAIL 40

North Fork Big Pine Creek Trail
Glacier Lodge Road

▲ Mt. Alice

△ Big Pine Creek

P

start & finish

Glacier Lodge

INYO

Big

Pine

Creek

NAT'L FOREST

South

Fork

Big

South Fork Big Pine Creek Tr.

● Willow Lake

Brainerd Lake

Finger Lake

JOHN MUIR

WILDERNESS

0   0.25   0.5   0.75   1 mile

0   0.25   0.5   0.75   1 kilometer

▲ Norman Clyde Peak

Middle
Palisade ▲

Middle Palisade
Glacier

▲ The Thumb

Disappointment
Peak ▲

N

KINGS CANYON NATIONAL PARK

Brainerd Lake

Alpinists from across the globe are drawn to the beauty and challenge of the bevy of 14,000-foot peaks known as the Palisades. Less adventurous recreationists can enjoy the splendid alpine scenery found in the Middle Palisades on this journey up the canyon of South Fork Big Pine Creek to Brainerd Lake and the off-trail backcountry beyond. Although the terrain is heavenly, parts of the ascent may seem to have less divine origins. The first half of the trip climbs reasonably on well-maintained tread but the second half climbs more steeply on rough and poorly maintained trail, which, at this altitude, may leave flatlanders perturbed and gasping for breath. Once at Brainerd Lake, the trials and tribulations are soon forgotten amid the overwhelming beauty. Those with off-trail ambitions can continue climbing to Finger Lake and an incredible view of the Middle Palisade Glacier.

Best Time

This is high alpine country. Consequently, trails don't shed their snow in these parts until midsummer, which is usually around mid-July following winters of average snowfall. Patches of snow may last into August in some years, especially on the north-facing slopes below the Palisades crest. Early August is generally the best time to see the wildflowers in bloom. September can be a fine time for a visit, but expect increasingly chilly nighttime temperatures as the month unfolds.

TRAIL USE
Dayhike, Backpack,
Run, Horse,
Dogs Allowed

LENGTH
10.0 miles, 5–6 hours

VERTICAL FEET
+3750/-700/±8900

DIFFICULTY
– 1 2 3 **4** 5 +

TRAIL TYPE
Out & Back

FEATURES
Mountain
Lake
Wildflowers
Great Views
Camping
Swimming
Fishing

FACILITIES
Campground
Resort

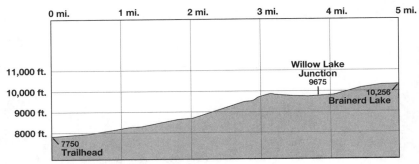

TRAIL 40 Brainerd Lake Elevation Profile

Finding the Trail

From U.S. Highway 395 in the center of Big Pine, turn west at Crocker Street and proceed out of town, as the road becomes Glacier Lodge Road. Follow the two-lane highway past campgrounds to the overnight parking area, or continue another three-quarters of a mile to the day-use lot near the end of the road. Both areas are equipped with vault toilets. The U.S. Forest Service administers three public campgrounds (fee, vault toilets, running water, bear boxes, and phone) along the Glacier Lodge Road, Upper Sage Flat, North Fork Big Pine, and Big Pine Creek. Two group campgrounds are also available by reservation. First Falls Walk-In is a no-fee campground for backpackers about a mile up the North Fork Trail, an excellent spot for those getting a late start. Although the main lodge building that housed a restaurant burned down a number of years ago, nearby Glacier Lodge continues to offer cabin rentals, guided trips, and pack trains.

Logistics

Backpackers must obtain a wilderness permit for all overnight visits. See page 238 for more details about how to obtain one.

Trail Description

▶1 From the day-use lot, stroll through shady forest next to Big Pine Creek along the continuation of the road past a few rustic cabins. Soon the road gives way to single-track trail, as you climb a forested hillside on rock steps and then proceed across a bridge spanning **North Fork Big Pine Creek**. Continue past the bridge to a junction with a connector to the **North Fork Trail**. ▶2

Bear left at the junction and cross an open, sagebrush-covered slope up the canyon of the cottonwood-lined South Fork Big Pine Creek, enjoying views of **Norman Clyde Peak** and **Middle Palisade** along the way. Cross over an old road and continue up-canyon on a moderate climb, crossing a seasonal stream and a boulder-filled slope on the way to a ford of the creek. A mild ascent heads away from the ford until a steep, winding climb via rocky switchbacks leads through scattered timber to the base of some nearly vertical bluffs. Traverse across the hillside and then climb steeply up a narrow cleft of rock to a crest and, after a short distance, a splendid panorama of the Palisades, stretching from **Mt. Sill** to **the Thumb**, a vista rivaling any in the Sierra for stunning alpine scenery. Past this splendid vista, the trail drops into the cover of lodgepole pines, passes a spring-fed rivulet, and then reaches a T-junction with a short lateral to **Willow Lake**. ▶3

The opal-tinted, icy waters of 10,256-foot Brainerd Lake are tucked into a deep, glacier-carved bowl of granite.

 Great Views

 Lake

Willow Lake

At 9565 feet, **Willow Lake** is just a short 0.3 mile jaunt away. Sediments are steadily transforming the lake into more of a marshy meadow, and in early summer, the standing water creates a haven for mosquitoes. However, a couple of lodgepole-shaded campsites offer overnight accommodations for backpackers who get a late start, or are too pooped to carry on toward Brainerd Lake.

OPTIONS

From the junction, a short descent heads down to a crossing of the lushly vegetated outlet from Brainerd Lake. From there, a winding ascent across a lodgepole-covered slope leads alongside the stream that drains Finger Lake. Turning east, the trail passes a small pond and continues uphill via switchbacks to a hump of granite that provides a fine view down-canyon of Willow Lake. Pass a second pond, make a short descent across a marshy meadow, and then swing around a granite ledge on a final climb south-east to the north shore of **Brainerd Lake**. ▶4

The opal-tinted, icy waters of 10,256-foot Brainerd Lake are tucked into a deep, glacier-carved bowl of granite. Steep cliffs hem in the lake on virtually all sides, with snow oftentimes lingering in narrow crevices late into the summer. The craggy, glacier-clad summits of the Palisades loom over the tops of the cliffs thousands of feet above. A smatter-

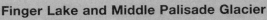

OPTIONS

Finger Lake and Middle Palisade Glacier

Without question the scenery around **Brainerd Lake** is stunning, but to come all this way and not go beyond the lake would be missing out on some even more extraordinary scenery. With a modicum of cross-country skills, hikers can quite easily make the short journey to slender Finger Lake by following a fairly well-defined, ducked use trail that begins near the outlet of Brainerd Lake. An arcing ascent leads above the cliffs on the northwest shore and then weaves through a boulder field to **Finger Lake**. The 10,787-foot lake nestled into a narrow cleft of rock that arcs toward the Palisades crest evokes a miniature Norwegian fjord. Scattered pines dot the lake-shore, while tiny pockets of wildflowers soften the otherwise stark surroundings. A few campsites can be found just below the lake between the outlet and the trail. To reach the edge of the glacier, head generally south from Finger Lake on a steep cross-country route up the canyon. The ascent can by physically taxing at this altitude, but the rewards of such dramatic alpine scenery more than compensate for the effort.

ing of compact campsites near the outlet, sheltered by lodgepole and whitebark pines, offer overnighters wonderfully scenic spots to rest their heads. Anglers may wish to test their luck on the brook trout that inhabit the lake.

Camping

Fishing

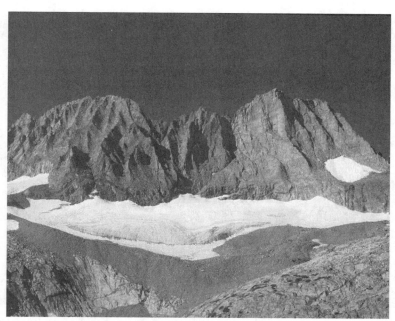

Middle Palisade and Disappointment Peak

🚶	**MILESTONES**

►1	0.0	Start at day-use trailhead
►2	0.3	Left at junction with connector to North Fork
►3	3.8	Ahead at Willow Lake junction
►4	5.0	Brainerd Lake

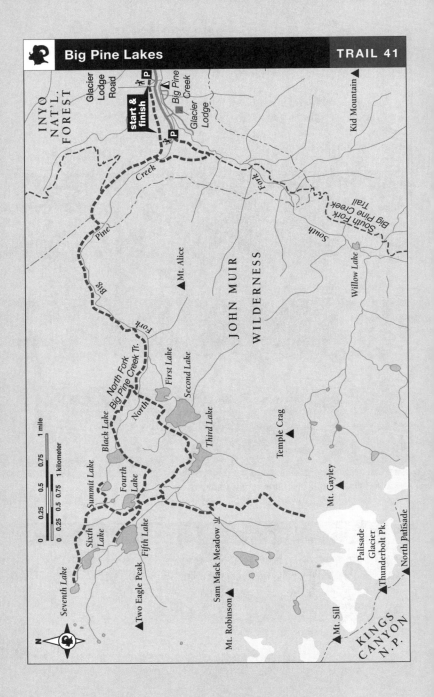

INYO NAT'L. FOREST

Glacier Lodge Road

P

Big Pine Creek

start & finish

Glacier Lodge

P

Kid Mountain

Creek

Fork

South Fork Big Pine Creek Trail

Pine

Big

Fork

North Fork Big Pine Creek Tr.

Mt. Alice

JOHN MUIR WILDERNESS

Willow Lake

First Lake

Second Lake

Third Lake

North

Black Lake

Summit Lake

Fourth Lake

Fifth Lake

Temple Crag

Mt. Gayley

Sixth Lake

Two Eagle Peak

Sam Mack Meadow

Mt. Robinson

Palisade Glacier

Thunderbolt Pk.

North Palisade

Seventh Lake

Mt. Sill

KINGS CANYON N.P.

1 mile

1 kilometer

0.25 0.5 0.75

0.25 0.5 0.75

0

N

Big Pine Lakes

Some of the best high alpine scenery in the Sierra can be found on this circuit through Big Pine Lakes basin in the North Fork Big Pine Creek drainage. Piercing the rarefied air near the upper height of the range, the group of peaks known as the Palisades compose a craggy spine of summits robed in scenic splendor as picturesque and dramatic as any in California, if not the entire western U.S. Clinging beneath the north face of these rugged peaks, a handful of glaciers, including the Palisade Glacier (the Sierra's largest), add a definite alpine ambiance to the area. Even the lower peaks, such as Temple Crag, cast a bold and rugged presence offering climbers a technical challenge and hikers a spectacular profile when viewed from a variety of vantage points along the trail. Nestled beneath the shadow of these towering peaks are the glacier-scoured basins holding the scenic Big Pine Lakes, the milky-turquoise color revealing the glacial origin of their waters. The shorelines of these lakes offer exceptional views of the surrounding wonders, as well as fine campsites.

Such spectacular scenery is bound to attract a large number of visitors, placing a high demand on the limited number of wilderness permits for those who desire to spend at least one night in the backcountry. As the trail climbs stiffly from the trailhead to the lake's basin, most overnighters seek campsites near the first lakes along the trail, allowing a higher possibility for solitude at the more far-flung lakes. Most dayhikers should find the 12.4-mile semiloop to be plenty challenging, but extremely strong hikers, as well as backpackers, will find trip extensions to lakes beyond the loop and to the Palisade Glacier well worth the extra time and energy.

TRAIL USE
Dayhike, Backpack,
Run, Horse,
Dogs Allowed

LENGTH
11.4 miles, 6–7 hours

VERTICAL FEET
+3175/-3175/±6350

DIFFICULTY
– 1 2 3 **4** 5 +

TRAIL TYPE
Semiloop

FEATURES
Mountain
Lake
Wildflowers
Great Views
Camping
Swimming
Historic Interest
Fishing

FACILITIES
Campground
Resort

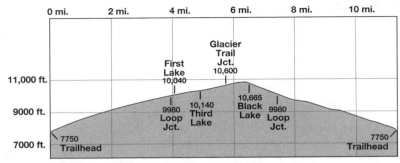

TRAIL 41 Big Pine Lakes Elevation Profile

Best Time

This is high alpine country. Consequently, trails don't shed their snow in these parts until midsummer, which is usually around mid-July following winters of average snowfall. Patches of snow may last into August in some years, especially on the north-facing slopes below the Palisades crest. Early August is generally the best time to see the wildflowers in bloom. September can be a fine time for a visit, but nighttime temperatures become increasingly chilly as the month unfolds.

Finding the Trail

From U.S. Highway 395 in the center of Big Pine, turn west at Crocker Street and proceed out of town, as the road becomes Glacier Lodge Road. Follow the two-lane highway past campgrounds to the overnight parking area, or continue another three-quarters of a mile to the day-use lot near the end of the road. Both areas are equipped with vault toilets. The U.S. Forest Service administers three public campgrounds (fee, vault toilets, running water, bear boxes, and phone) along the Glacier Lodge Road, Upper Sage Flat, North Fork Big Pine, and Big Pine Creek. Two group campgrounds are also available by reservation. First Falls Walk-In is a no-fee campground for backpackers about a mile up the North Fork Trail, an excellent spot for those getting a late start. Although the main lodge building that housed a restaurant burned down a number of years ago, nearby Glacier Lodge continues to offer cabin rentals, guided trips, and pack trains.

Logistics

Backpackers must obtain a wilderness permit for all overnight visits. See page 238 for more details about how to obtain one.

Trail Description

▶1 From the day-use lot, stroll through shady forest next to **Big Pine Creek** along the continuation of the road past a few rustic cabins. Soon the road gives way to single-track trail, as you climb a forested hillside on rock steps and then proceed across a bridge spanning **North Fork Big Pine Creek**. Continue past the bridge to a junction with your connector to the **North Fork Trail**. ▶2

Bear right at the junction and follow short switchbacks up an open slope with good views up the South Fork canyon. Back under shady forest, the grade eases on the way to a T-junction with an old road. ▶3 Turn right and proceed a short distance on the roadbed to a bridge over the creek and shortly to another junction. ▶4 Following a sign marked UPPER TRAIL, veer right away from the road and head east-southeast, climbing steeply, then more gradually to a junction ▶5 with the trail from the overnight parking lot. Along the way, fine views of the long cascade of Second Falls should cheer you onward.

Turn left and ascend open slopes toward Second Falls. After some switchbacks, you cross into **John Muir Wilderness** and head up a chasm. Above the falls, the trail climbs moderately alongside the

The shorelines of these lakes offer exceptional views of the surrounding wonders, as well as fine campsites.

Lon Chaney Cabin

HISTORY

In what appears to be the middle of nowhere sits a distinguished granite fieldstone cabin with gable roof and overhanging eaves. Used nowadays by rangers as a wilderness cabin, the structure was originally built at the behest of silent film star Lon Chaney in the 1920s. Chaney used the cabin as a summer retreat, where he relaxed, fished, and hunted. Listed on the National Register of Historic Places, the cabin was designed by Paul Revere Williams, who holds the distinction of being the first African-American granted a fellowship by the American Institute of Architects.

shady creek for a spell, wanders back out into the open, and then follows gently graded tread across an aspen- and lodgepole-shaded flat known as Cienega Mirth (a combination of a misspelled Spanish word and a Scottish word, both meaning swampy place). A number of pleasant campsites are spread about this flat.

Beyond **Lon Chaney's cabin**, the trail passes through an open area with a glimpse of some of the ragged peaks at the head of the canyon. The moderate ascent resumes, as the trail wanders back and forth to the creek several times through lush vegetation and light forest. Where the trail bends west, the dramatic northeast face of Temple Crag makes brief appearances. Cross willow-lined **North Fork Big Pine Creek**, climb more steeply via switchbacks, and then cross back over the creek, beyond which more climbing leads to a junction with the beginning of the loop section. ▶6

Follow the left-hand trail, signed LAKES 1–7, immediately cross the creek, pass a couple of campsites, and keep climbing through scattered forest and granite slabs and around large boulders. The sound of running water from a cascade heralds the presence of nearby **First Lake**, ▶7 its milky-turquoise, glacier-fed waters visible through gaps in the forest. Farther on, a zigzagging descent leads to a spectacular over-look of **Second Lake**, with an impressive backdrop from the towering ramparts of 12,999-foot Temple Crag. Although Second Lake is the largest in the chain of Big Pine Lakes, much of the shoreline is too steep to allow decent camping. Although a few isolated campsites can be found spread around the shoreline, most backpackers are more content with sites above the west shore of First Lake. Anglers can practice their craft on brook, brown, and rainbow trout in both lakes. Mildly graded trail leads well above the surface of Second Lake, where sparse forest permits stunning views of the surrounding terrain.

Beyond Second Lake, the trail follows the inlet on a climb through rocky terrain beneath a cover of lodgepole pines, before veering away from the stream on the way to the north shore of Third Lake. ▶8 Here's an even more impressive view of Temple Crag, perhaps the main reason backpackers pre-fer the numerous campsites sprinkled around the lightly forested shoreline. Anglers may be tempted by the brook and rainbow trout seen gliding through the chilly waters.

 Lake

 Camping

 Fishing

 Camping

Grand Views

The stunning views from the trail above Second Lake include the dramatic and precipitous flying buttresses of Temple Crag, rising high above the crystalline water. Challenging Class 5 routes on **Temple Crag** lure climbers from around the world. In stark con-trast, the massive rock pile to the east, Mt. Alice, has been dubbed "one of the ugliest peaks in the Sierra—a veritable pile of rubble" by author Steve Roper, who expressed his disdain for the peak in *Climbers Guide to the High Sierra*. Separating these two peaks is **Contact Pass**, where the line between the darker and lighter shades of granite is quite evident. The pass provides a cross-country route between the two canyons of Big Pine Creek.

Palisade Glacier Trail

The steep 2-mile, 1600-foot climb to the **Palisade Glacier** may be well beyond the reach of most day-trippers, but those with extra time and energy will be well rewarded for the effort with absolutely outstanding scenery. From the junction, turn left and head southwest through a willow-covered meadow and across a stream draining Fifth Lake, before a zigzagging climb leads up a rocky slope through widely scattered whitebark pines. Midway up the slope is a luxuriant, spring-fed grotto carpeted with abundant wildflowers. Farther up the hillside, the path ascends alongside the creek, which is lined with more flowers, including paintbrush, buttercup, shooting star, daisy, aster, and columbine. Where the grade eases, you crest the lip of the basin holding beautiful **Sam Mack Meadow** and proceed across the long, thin meadowland bordered by steep walls of gray granite and bisected by a sinuous brook tinged with white glacial milk. Snow clings to the precipitous walls at the head of the canyon, lingering throughout the short summers common at this elevation. A few campsites perched on a sloping, sandy bench adjacent to the meadow and shaded by clumps of dwarf pines may tempt overnighters. Although a footpath extends to the far end of the meadow, Sam Mack Lake is most easily reached by heading cross-country up the west canyon wall and then southwest to the lakeshore.

To continue toward Palisade Glacier, ford the creek near the lower end of the meadow, where an old, small sign simply marked TRAIL points the way across the broad but shallow brook to a use trail on the far side that ascends the east wall of the canyon. Wind up the rocky hillside to the crest and then turn south, continuing to wind around boulders and rocks amid widely scattered whitebark pines up the left-hand side of a ridge, with excellent views down to **Big Pine Lakes**. About a mile from Sam Mack Meadow, the route bends southeast and follows an ascending traverse to a moraine. The path becomes less discernible, as you climb more steeply across talus, boulders, and slabs, but ducks should help to keep you on track. The tread completely disappears at an overlook of the **Palisade Glacier**, from where fortunate visitors enjoy a splendid view of the jagged Palisades.

Switchbacks lead away from **Third Lake** on a climb out of the lake's basin. Take the time to look behind you, as the view of Third Lake reposing in a rocky bowl at the base of Temple Crag and the craggy summits of **the Palisades** is quite impressive, along with the massive face of Mt. Robinson and Aperture Peak just behind. The grade eases a bit near a small meadow, where you hop across a tiny rivulet that drains **Fourth Lake**. Just beyond this rivulet is a junction near a grove of pines with the **Glacier Trail**. ▶9

From the Glacier Trail junction, head northwest on a moderate climb through scattered pines and past rocks and boulders, with pleasant views of the Palisades to a four-way junction. ▶10 The left-hand trail leads a quarter mile to Fifth Lake, while the trail straight ahead provides access to Sixth and Seventh lakes.

To continue to **Fifth Lake**, turn left from the junction and proceed through light forest to the lake's outlet. Continue alongside the willow-lined creek on gently graded tread to the east shore of the picturesque lake, where rugged mountains, including Mt. Robinson, Two Eagle Peak, and Aperture Peak, form a scenic arc around the sapphire waters. The more distant summits of **Temple Crag, Mt. Gayley, Mt. Sill**, and **the Inconsolable Range** provide additional visual delight. A smattering of pines dot the shoreline and the lower slopes of the basin, while grasses, sedges, and shrubs carpet the small pockets of soil between the rocky cliffs and talus slopes. Pleasant campsites near the inlet and farther around the shoreline will tempt overnighters.

Back at the four-way junction with the trail to **Sixth and Seventh lakes**, head northwest above the west shore of Fourth Lake to continue to the other lakes and then ascend a low hill past some campsites. The grade increases where you cross a willow-lined stream flowing into Fourth Lake. Near

 Great Views

 Camping

 Camping

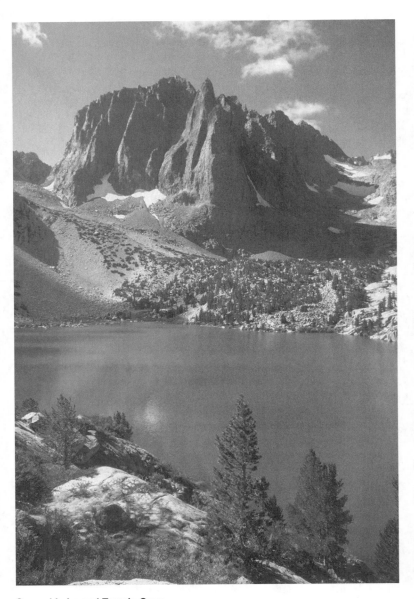

Second Lake and Temple Crag

the stream an old and obscure path heads northwest to Sixth Lake, but the path soon deteriorates
to more of a cross-country route. Traveling in the
opposite direction leads very shortly to a level spot
on a ridge with some campsites and an incredible
view of the Palisades, spanning from Temple Crag Great Views
to Mt. Winchell. This excellent view was the reason
the Fourth Lake Lodge was built here in the 1920s.
The Forest Service removed the lodge and eight
cabins after passage of the original Wilderness Act
of 1964. Continue ahead from the stream to a junction, where the left-hand branch continues to Sixth
and Seventh lakes, and the right-hand trail provides
access to Summit Lake.

Turn left (north) and continue toward **Sixth
Lake**, climbing moderately steeply on rocky switchbacks; the climb is briefly interrupted where you
stroll past a pond surrounded by a small meadow.
Reach the top of a lightly forested rise, with a good
view of the Palisades just off the trail, and then drop
off the rise to the crossing of a stream in a meadow.
From there, a short climb over a rock hump leads
to a smaller meadow, followed by a short climb
into Sixth Lake's basin. A brief descent brings you
to the southeast shore. With meadows surrounding
the lake and low rises dotted with whitebark pines
edging the meadows, the ambiance around Sixth
Lake is much more pastoral than at the other Big
Pine Lakes. The open terrain allows good views of
Mt. Robinson, Two Eagle Peak, and **Cloudripper,**
as well as the more distant **Temple Crag** and **Mt.
Gayley**. Backpackers will find decent campsites Camping
scattered about the low rises around the lake.

Although no maintained trail exists between
Sixth and Seventh lakes, the route is straightforward across open meadowlands dotted with clumps
of willow; simply head west-northwest along the
course of the stream connecting the two lakes for a
quarter mile to the east shore of **Seventh Lake**. The

lake is quite pleasant, tucked into an open basin below the slopes of Cloudripper. The few campsites sprinkled above the lakeshore seem to be more than adequate for the small number of campers who visit the lake.

 Camping

Summit Lake can be reached by retracing your steps to the junction between the trails to Sixth Lake and Summit Lake. Turn left and climb moderately to the crest of a ridge, where the lake suddenly appears through the trees. A short descent leads to the roughly oval, forest-lined lake, perched on a bench above a steep drop toward Black Lake below. Campsites seem plentiful and anglers can test their skills on the resident brook trout.

Camping

Fishing

From the four-way junction, ►10 the loop portion of the trip continues by turning northeast and skirting the south shore of **Fourth Lake**. Gently descending trail through scattered to light forest is followed by a gentle ascent over a forested rise and a moderate descent through lodgepole pines to the south shore of **Black Lake**. ►11 A number of fine campsites around the lake and above the trail offer potential overnight havens. Anglers can ply the waters in search of brook and rainbow trout.

Fishing

A steep descent leads away from Black Lake, as you eventually break out of the forest to views of **Mt. Alice** and **Temple Crag** across the North Fork canyon, and **Mt. Sill** and **North Palisade** along the crest. Farther along, several of the Big Pine Lakes spring into view. Long-legged switchbacks lead across a sagebrush-covered slope dotted with mountain mahogany, wild rose, and an occasional whitebark or lodgepole pine. Reach the close of the loop about a mile from Black Lake ►12 and then retrace your steps to the parking lot. ►13

 Great Views

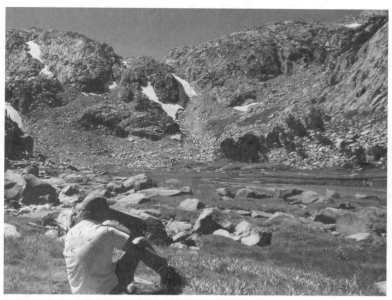

Sam Mack Meadow *on the Palisade Glacier Trail*

🚶 MILESTONES

►1	0.0	Start at day-use trailhead
►2	0.3	Right at connector junction
►3	0.4	Right at road
►4	0.5	Right to Upper Trail
►5	0.7	Left at Upper Trail
►6	3.9	Left at loop junction
►7	4.1	First Lake
►8	4.9	Third Lake
►9	5.7	Glacier Trail junction
►10	5.9	Right at Fifth Lake junction
►11	6.6	Black Lake
►12	7.5	Left at loop junction
►13	11.4	Return to trailhead

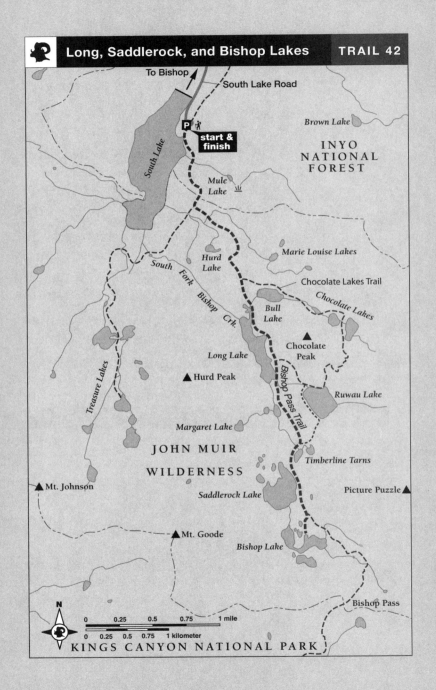

To Bishop

South Lake Road

P

start & finish

South Lake

Brown Lake

INYO
NATIONAL
FOREST

Mule
Lake

Marie Louise Lakes

Hurd
Lake

Chocolate Lakes Trail

South Fork Bishop Crk.

Chocolate Lakes

Bull
Lake

Chocolate
Peak

Long Lake

▲ Hurd Peak

Ruwau Lake

Treasure Lakes

Bishop Pass Trail

Margaret Lake

JOHN MUIR

Timberline Tarns

WILDERNESS

▲ Mt. Johnson

Picture Puzzle ▲

Saddlerock Lake

▲ Mt. Goode

Bishop Lake

N

0   0.25   0.5   0.75   1 mile

0 0.25 0.5 0.75 1 kilometer

Bishop Pass

KINGS CANYON NATIONAL PARK

Long, Saddlerock, and Bishop Lakes

The terrain in the upper reaches of South Fork Bishop Creek drainage is highly popular with a wide range of recreationists, making securing a wilderness permit or a parking place a dubious proposition on summer weekends. Unless you're willing to step off the trail, solitude is an elusive commodity. Nonetheless, a bounty of picturesque lakes, rugged peaks, rushing streams, vibrant wildflowers, verdant meadows, and groves of pines all lure you to this classic eastern Sierra journey. Adding a 2.5-mile side excursion to the Chocolate Lakes creates a fine semiloop trip (see Trail 44).

Best Time

The South Fork Bishop Creek drainage tends to shed most of its snow by early July and wildflowers reach their peak from mid-July into early August. The water temperature of these high mountain lakes is always a bit chilly, but swimmers will find the conditions at their best from mid- to late August. Late summer and early autumn can be a great time for a trip, when the crowds have diminished and the weather is cooler but usually sunny. By late October or early November the area has usually seen the first significant storm of the season.

Finding the Trail

Turn west from U.S. Highway 395 in the center of Bishop at Line Drive, and proceed out of town, as the road becomes South Lake Road (Highway 168). Proceed 15 miles to a junction and turn left toward

TRAIL USE
Dayhike, Backpack,
Run, Horse,
Dogs Allowed

LENGTH
8.6 miles, 4–5 hours

VERTICAL FEET
+1750/-250/±4000

DIFFICULTY
– 1 2 **3** 4 5 +

TRAIL TYPE
Out & Back

FEATURES
Mountain
Lake
Wildflowers
Camping
Swimming
Fishing

FACILITIES
Campground
Resort

301

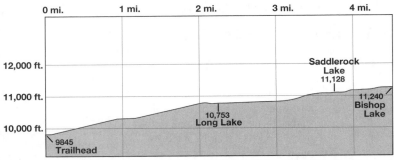

0 mi. 1 mi. 2 mi. 3 mi. 4 mi.

12,000 ft.

Saddlerock
Lake
11,128

11,000 ft.

11,240
Bishop
Lake

10,753
Long Lake

10,000 ft.

9845
Trailhead

TRAIL 42 Long, Saddlerock, and Bishop Lakes Elevation Profile

Nestled in a glacier-scoured basin at the foot of the towering northeast buttress of Mt. Goode, Saddlerock Lake offers an austere haven for backpackers.

South Lake. Continue another 6.75 miles to the end of the road near the South Lake Dam. Backpackers must park in the overnight lot—when this lot is full, additional overnight parking is usually available 1.3 miles back down the road near Parchers Resort (a footpath connects the upper and lower lots). Day-use parking is available just below the overnight lot. Vault toilets and water are available nearby. Four Forest Service campgrounds are located along South Lake Road, Forks (fee, flush toilets, running water, and phone) Four Jeffrey (fee, flush toilets, and running water), Mountain Glen (vault toilets and fee), and Willow (vault toilets and fee). Resorts strung along South Lake Road include Bishop Creek Lodge, Cardinal Village Resort, and Parchers Resort.

Logistics

Backpackers must obtain a wilderness permit for all overnight visits. See page 238 for more details about how to obtain one.

Trail Description

►1 The well-marked trail begins near the south end of the overnight parking lot, immediately making a very short and steep descent through lush trailside

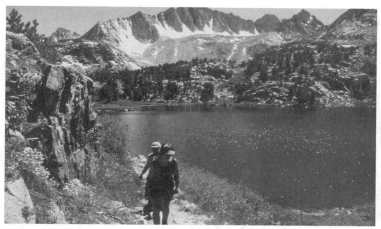

Hiking *along Long Lake with Mt. Goode in the background*

vegetation. A mild climb leads well above the east shore of South Lake through young aspens and lodgepole pines before the trail breaks out into the open to fine views up-canyon of South Fork Bishop Creek. Soon a steeper ascent heads up the hillside past the **John Muir Wilderness boundary** and to a Y-junction with the **Treasure Lakes Trail.** ▶2 Veer to the left and head southeast through light lodgepole pine forest to a plank bridge across a small, flower-lined stream, followed by a moderate climb to an unmarked junction with the partly cross-country route to the seldom-visited **Marie Louise Lakes.** Just past this faint junction, you briefly come alongside and cross another small creek before climbing over granite outcrops and around boulders via switchbacks to a Y-junction with the lower end of the **Chocolate Lakes Trail.** ▶3

Wildflowers

Remaining on the **Bishop Pass Trail**, an easy quarter-mile stroll leads over to the north shore of aptly named **Long Lake**. The elongated lake is bordered by verdant green meadows, granite boulders, and scattered conifers. Tiny islets sprinkle the crystal-blue waters, which reflect the craggy images

Chocolate Lakes Loop

Returning to the trailhead via the **Chocolate Lakes Trail** is a fairly straightforward endeavor, adding a mere 2.5 miles to the journey. Although returning to the upper loop junction near the south end of Long Lake is the most apparent way, the cross-country route from Timberline Tarns is more direct. From the easternmost tarn, ascend north over a low bench and drop down to scenic **Ruwau Lake**, sandwiched between Chocolate Peak and the Inconsolable Range. Pick up maintained trail on the north shore and climb deteriorating tread up and over the divide separating Ruwau Lake from the Chocolate Lakes. Drop down to the **three Chocolate Lakes** and then **Bull Lake** before descending steeply to the lower junction below the north end of Long Lake. From there, retrace your steps 1.9 miles to the trailhead.

Camping

Lake

Wildflowers

Camping

of Mt. Goode and Hurd Peak. Lovely scenery, close proximity to a trailhead, and a healthy population of rainbow, brook, and brown trout make this lake a very popular destination for hikers, backpackers, and anglers. Campsites abound around the overused shoreline, especially on a knoll near the south end of the lake. As you continue up the trail along the east shore, Long Lake seems to go on forever. Reach a T-junction ▶4 with the upper end of the **Chocolate Lakes Trail** near the far end of the lake.

From the junction, proceed ahead a short distance along the south end of Long Lake, cross the inlet from **Ruwau Lake**, and then resume the climb through a light to scattered forest of whitebark pines. Continue climbing through small meadows, fields of rock, and pockets of wildflowers to the east of picturesque **Spearhead Lake**, backdropped by the spine of the Inconsolable Range. Limited campsites are scattered around the shore, and fishing is reported to be fair for rainbow and brook trout.

Straightforward cross-country travel leads west from the lake to lovely and isolated **Margaret Lake**.

 Lake

A half-mile climb from Spearhead Lake on the Bishop Pass Trail ascends a rocky slope to the lovely **Timberline Tarns**, where sparkling waterfalls and tumbling cascades greet you along the way. While most backpackers bypass this area in favor of campsites at the larger lakes above, a handful of fine, out-of-the-way sites nearby are worthwhile overnight havens. An easy cross-country route from the easternmost tarn heads north over a low bench to Ruwau Lake.

 Camping

From Timberline Tarns, a short climb leads to the east shore of island-dotted **Saddlerock Lake**. ▶5 Nestled in a glacier-scoured basin at the foot of the towering northeast buttress of Mt. Goode, the lake offers an austere haven for backpackers. Anglers can ply the waters in search of the elusive rainbow and brook trout.

 Fishing

As the Bishop Pass Trail avoids Bishop Lake, an unmarked use trail from Saddlerock Lake heading south over a low rise is the preferred route to irregular-shaped **Bishop Lake**. ▶6 Good campsites can be found on the low rise just north of the lake. Rainbow and brook trout are also present in Bishop Lake.

 Camping

🚶	**MILESTONES**		
▶1	0.0	Start at trailhead
▶2	0.75	Straight at Treasure Lakes junction
▶3	1.9	Straight at Lower Chocolate Lakes junction
▶4	2.7	Straight at Upper Chocolate Lakes junction
▶5	3.75	Saddlerock Lake
▶6	4.3	Bishop Lake

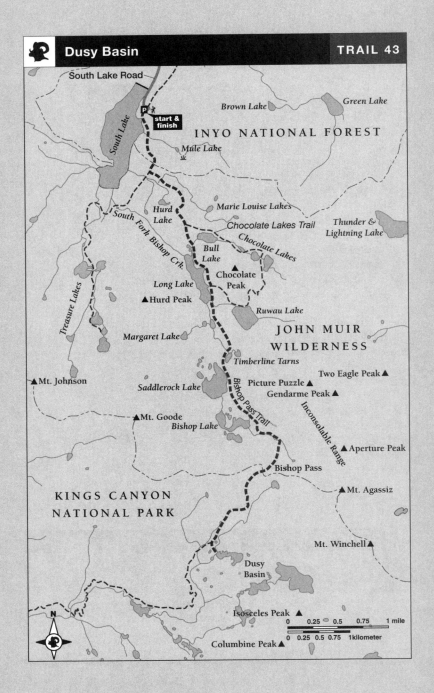

South Lake Road

Brown Lake

Green Lake

P

start & finish

INYO NATIONAL FOREST

Mule Lake

South Lake

Hurd Lake

Marie Louise Lakes

South Fork Bishop Crk.

Chocolate Lakes Trail

Thunder & Lightning Lake

Bull Lake

Chocolate Lakes

Chocolate Peak

Long Lake

Treasure Lakes

▲Hurd Peak

Ruwau Lake

Margaret Lake

JOHN MUIR WILDERNESS

Timberline Tarns

▲Mt. Johnson

Saddlerock Lake

Picture Puzzle ▲

Two Eagle Peak ▲

Gendarme Peak ▲

Bishop Pass Trail

▲Mt. Goode

Bishop Lake

Inconsolable Range

▲Aperture Peak

Bishop Pass

KINGS CANYON

NATIONAL PARK

▲ Mt. Agassiz

Mt. Winchell▲

Dusy Basin

N

Isosceles Peak ▲

0   0.25   0.5   0.75   1 mile

0   0.25 0.5 0.75   1 kilometer

Columbine Peak ▲

Dusy Basin

Dusy Basin is one of the most scenic areas in the High Sierra, where picturesque tarns encircled by lush meadows and sparkling granite slabs contrast vividly with an amphitheater of classic alpine peaks. Although the basin lies a mere 7.5 miles from a trailhead, the rugged climb over nearly 12,000-foot-high Bishop Pass is enough of a physical challenge to deter at least a percentage of the area's worshippers. Many backpackers require two days just to reach Dusy Basin, taking the trip out of the realm of a two-day weekend for most, but this is not necessarily detrimental, as the area is so beautiful that hikers could spend many extra days exploring all its nooks and crannies.

Best Time

As snow tends to linger on the north slope below Bishop Pass well into summer, trail users hoping for snow-free tread should wait until August in years following an average winter. Those who don't mind traversing a little snow can generally get over the pass by mid-July without too much trouble. Dusy Basin is typically in full regalia from late July into early August, when wildflowers add a riot of color, meadow grasses are deep green, and rivulets are flowing with sparkling water (unfortunately, mosquitoes also peak during this time). Fair weather usually extends well into September, but backpackers should be prepared for chilly nighttime temperatures as the month progresses. The first storm of the season usually visits the region by late October or early November.

TRAIL USE
Dayhike, Backpack, Run

LENGTH
15.2 miles, 8 hours

VERTICAL FEET
+2500/-1550/±8100

DIFFICULTY
- 1 2 3 **4** 5 +

TRAIL TYPE
Out & Back

FEATURES
Mountain
Lake
Wildflowers
Great Views
Camping
Swimming
Fishing

FACILITIES
Campground
Resort

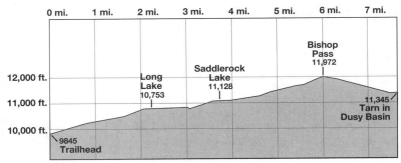

TRAIL 43 Dusy Basin Elevation Profile

Finding the Trail

Turn west from U.S. Highway 395 in the center of Bishop at Line Drive, and proceed out of town, as the road becomes South Lake Road (Highway 168). Proceed 15 miles to a junction and turn left toward South Lake. Continue another 6.75 miles to the end of the road near the South Lake Dam. Backpackers must park in the overnight lot—when this lot is full, additional overnight parking is usually available 1.3 miles back down the road near Parchers Resort (a footpath connects the upper and lower lots). Day-use parking is available just below the overnight lot. Vault toilets and water are available nearby. Four Forest Service campgrounds are located along South Lake Road, Forks (fee, flush toilets, running water, and phone) Four Jeffrey (fee, flush toilets, and running water), Mountain Glen (vault toilets and fee), and Willow (vault toilets and fee). Resorts strung along South Lake Road include Bishop Creek Lodge, Cardinal Village Resort, and Parchers Resort.

Logistics

Backpackers must obtain a wilderness permit for all overnight visits. See page 238 for more details about how to obtain one.

Trail Description

▶1 The well-marked trail begins near the south end of the overnight parking lot, immediately making a very short and steep descent through lush trailside vegetation. A mild climb leads well above the east shore of South Lake through young aspens and lodgepole pines before the trail breaks out into the open to fine views up-canyon of South Fork Bishop Creek. Soon a steeper ascent heads up the hillside past the **John Muir Wilderness boundary** and to a Y-junction with the **Treasure Lakes Trail**. ▶2 Veer to the left and head southeast through light lodge-pole pine forest to a plank bridge across a small, flower-lined stream, followed by a moderate climb to an unmarked junction with the partly cross-country route to the seldom-visited Marie Louise Lakes. Just past this faint junction, you briefly come alongside and cross another small creek and then climb over granite outcrops and around boulders via switchbacks to a Y-junction with the lower end of the **Chocolate Lakes Trail**. ▶3

Remaining on the **Bishop Pass Trail**, an easy quarter-mile stroll leads over to the north shore of aptly named **Long Lake**. The elongated lake is bordered by verdant green meadows, granite boulders, and scattered conifers. Tiny islets sprinkle the crystal-blue waters, which reflect the craggy images of Mt. Goode and Hurd Peak. The lovely scenery combined with the close proximity to the trailhead and a healthy population of rainbow, brook, and brown trout make the lake a very popular destination for hikers, backpackers, and anglers. Campsites abound around the overused shoreline, especially on a knoll near the south end of the lake. As you continue up the trail along the east shore, Long Lake seems to go on forever. Reach a T-junction ▶4 with the upper end of the **Chocolate Lakes Trail** near the far end of the lake.

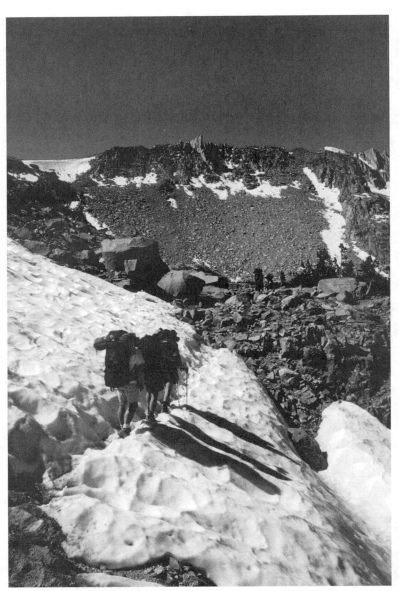

Climbing toward Bishop Pass

From the junction, proceed ahead a short distance along the south end of Long Lake, cross the inlet from **Ruwau Lake**, and then resume the climb through a light to scattered forest of whitebark pines. Continue climbing through small meadows, fields of rock, and pockets of wildflowers to the east of picturesque **Spearhead Lake**, backdropped by the spine of the Inconsolable Range. Limited campsites are scattered around the shore, and fishing is reported to be fair for rainbow and brook trout. Straightforward cross-country travel leads west from the lake to lovely and isolated **Margaret Lake**.

 Wildflowers

A half-mile climb from Spearhead Lake on the Bishop Pass Trail ascends a rocky slope to the lovely **Timberline Tarns**, where sparkling waterfalls and tumbling cascades greet you along the way. While most backpackers bypass this area in favor of campsites at the larger lakes above, a handful of fine, out-of-the-way sites nearby are worthwhile overnight havens. An easy cross-country route from the easternmost tarn heads north over a low bench to Ruwau Lake.

 Camping

From Timberline Tarns, a short climb leads to the east shore of island-dotted **Saddlerock Lake**. ▶5 Nestled in a glacier-scoured basin at the foot of the towering northeast buttress of Mt. Goode, the lake offers an austere haven for backpackers. Anglers can ply the waters in search of the elusive rainbow and brook trout.

 Lake
 Camping

Dusy Basin

Dusy Basin was named for a Canadian-born shepherd, Frank Dusy, who drove his flocks into the Kings River backcountry, exploring the Middle Fork all the way into the Palisades. He is credited with the discovery of remote Tehipite Valley in 1869, photographing the area for the first time 10 years later.

Continuing up the Bishop Pass Trail, you pass timberline and enter the alpine zone on rocky tread composed of red, metamorphic rock. Soon the grade increases, as the rock type switches back to the characteristic Sierra granite. Climb the impressive canyon headwall via winding trail toward Bishop Pass through a seemingly endless sea of boulders and slabs and, depending on the season, patches of snow. While catching your breath at rest stops, you can enjoy the spectacular views of Mt. Goode and the jagged spires of the Inconsolable Range. Eventually you reach **Bishop Pass**, ►6 where the view of the tarns and meadowlands of **Dusy Basin** backdropped by Giraud and Columbine peaks is quite striking. To the southwest, beyond the deep chasm of LeConte Canyon, the **Black Divide** casts a regal profile slicing across the deep blue sky. Flanking the pass to the northeast, **Mt. Aggasiz** beckons energetic peakbaggers on a scramble toward the summit.

> Dusy Basin is an exquisitely beautiful area, with azure-tinted tarns rimmed by pockets of luxuriant meadow and bordered by sparkling granite slabs.

After the taxing uphill stretch to Bishop Pass, sandy tread descends to some switchbacks, where a fairly well-defined use trail travels shortly above the main trail to the top of a cliff and an excellent view of Dusy Basin and the surrounding peaks and ridges. Back on the main trail, continue winding downhill past welcome patches of green meadow, pockets of wildflowers, and some gurgling meltwater rivulets—at least until later in the season, when the rivulets dry up, the flowers fade, and the meadows turn golden. Along the descent, you experience fine views of Dusy Basin's numerous tarns and pocket meadows, dramatically framed by the craggy **Palisades and Isosceles and Columbine peaks**. Approximately 1.5 miles from Bishop Pass, a use trail branches away from the main trail to the left, leading to the uppermost tarn ►7 in the basin. Although several campsites are located around the shoreline, more secluded sites may be found around the tarns farther east.

 Great Views

 Camping

Dusy Basin is an exquisitely beautiful area, with azure-tinted tarns rimmed by pockets of luxuriant meadow and bordered by sparkling granite slabs. In early season, tiny ribbons of crystalline brooks refresh the meadows and pour into the tarns. No matter what the season, rugged spires pierce the rarified air and precipitous faces tantalize even the most casual mountain lover. The delicate alpine vegetation in the basin is quite fragile, so backpackers should locate their camps only in areas of sandy soil. While the open nature of the basin is well suited to cross-country travel, off-trail enthusiasts should minimize their impact on the fragile plant life. Anglers can fish for golden and brook trout.

 Fishing

🚶	**MILESTONES**

►1	0.0	Start at trailhead
►2	0.75	Straight at Treasure Lakes Trail junction
►3	1.9	Straight at lower Chocolate Lakes Trail junction
►4	2.7	Straight at upper Chocolate Lakes Trail junction
►5	3.75	Saddlerock Lake
►6	6.0	Bishop Pass
►7	7.6	Uppermost tarn in Dusy Basin

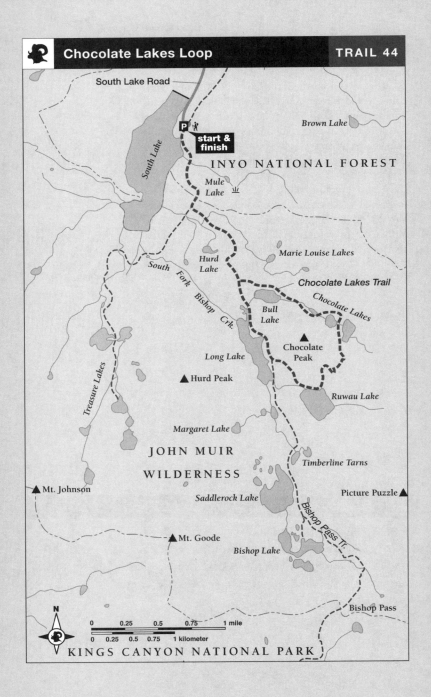

South Lake Road

P

start & finish

Brown Lake

INYO NATIONAL FOREST

South Lake

Mule Lake

Hurd Lake

Marie Louise Lakes

South Fork Bishop Crk.

Chocolate Lakes Trail

Chocolate Lakes

Bull Lake

Treasure Lakes

Long Lake

▲ Hurd Peak

▲ Chocolate Peak

Ruwau Lake

Margaret Lake

JOHN MUIR

WILDERNESS

Timberline Tarns

▲ Mt. Johnson

Picture Puzzle ▲

Saddlerock Lake

▲ Mt. Goode

Bishop Lake

Bishop Pass Tr.

N

0   0.25   0.5   0.75   1 mile

0   0.25   0.5   0.75   1 kilometer

Bishop Pass

KINGS CANYON NATIONAL PARK

Chocolate Lakes Loop

The short semiloop around aptly named Chocolate Peak branches off the well-traveled Bishop Pass Trail to a string of picturesque lakes. Additional rewards include not only some outstanding scenery but also a sense of relative seclusion away from the steady stream of hikers, backpackers, and equestrians headed up the canyon of South Fork Bishop Creek. Unfortunately, backpackers seeking to overnight at the Chocolate Lakes have to compete for the same number of permits issued for those bound for the more popular destinations along the Bishop Pass Trail. However the 7.2-mile distance is well suited to dayhiking, which doesn't require a permit. Sections of the trail between Chocolate Lakes and Ruwau Lake are rough—indistinct in parts and indiscernible in others—although route-finding is straightforward. Anglers may find the fishing to be quite good.

TRAIL USE
Dayhike, Backpack,
Run, Horse,
Dogs Allowed

LENGTH
7.2 miles, 3–4 hours

VERTICAL FEET
+1690/-1690/±3380

DIFFICULTY
– 1 2 **3** 4 5 +

TRAIL TYPE
Semiloop

FEATURES
Mountain
Lake
Wildflowers
Camping
Swimming
Fishing

FACILITIES
Campground
Resort

Best Time

Trail users can usually follow a snow-free trail around the Chocolate Lakes as early as the first part of July. Wildflowers should be at their peak from mid-July through early August.

Finding the Trail

Turn west from U.S. Highway 395 in the center of Bishop at Line Drive, and proceed out of town, as the road becomes South Lake Road (Highway 168). Proceed 15 miles to a junction and turn left toward South Lake. Continue another 6.75 miles to the end

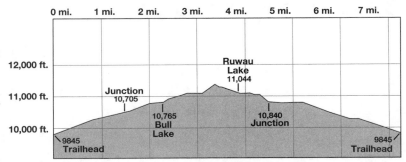

TRAIL 44 Chocolate Lakes Loop Elevation Profile

of the road near the South Lake Dam. Backpackers must park in the overnight lot—when this lot is full, additional overnight parking is usually available 1.3 miles back down the road near Parchers Resort (a footpath connects the upper and lower lots). Day-use parking is available just below the overnight lot. Vault toilets and water are available nearby. Four Forest Service campgrounds are located along South Lake Road, Forks (fee, flush toilets, running water, and phone) Four Jeffrey (fee, flush toilets, and running water), Mountain Glen (vault toilets and fee), and Willow (vault toilets and fee). Resorts strung along South Lake Road include Bishop Creek Lodge, Cardinal Village Resort, and Parchers Resort.

Logistics

Backpackers must obtain a wilderness permit for all overnight visits. See page 238 for more details about how to obtain one.

Trail Description

►1 The well-marked trail begins near the south end of the overnight parking lot, immediately making a very short and steep descent through lush trailside vegetation. A mild climb leads well above the east shore of South Lake through young aspens and lodgepole pines before the trail breaks out into the open to fine views up the canyon of South Fork Bishop Creek. Soon a steeper ascent heads up the hillside past the **John Muir Wilderness boundary** and to a Y-junction with the **Treasure Lakes Trail**. ▶2 Veer to the left and head southeast through light lodgepole pine forest to a plank bridge across a small, flower-lined stream, followed by a moderate climb to an unmarked junction with the partly cross-country route to the seldom-visited **Marie Louise Lakes**. Just past this faint junction, you briefly come alongside and cross another small creek before climbing over granite outcrops and around boulders via switchbacks to a Y-junction with the lower end of the **Chocolate Lakes Trail**. ▶3

Turn left at the junction, cross a talus slide, and ascend a steep draw to a meadow, soon arriving at **Bull Lake**. ▶4 The shoreline of the picturesque lake is blanketed with a light forest of whitebark pines, wildflowers, and scattered clumps of willow. Plenty of decent campsites are just off the trail. Anglers can test their skill on the resident brook trout.

The trail proceeds around the north shore of Bull Lake, crosses the inlet, and then climbs moderately steeply alongside the inlet through a fine display of wildflowers, including columbine, shooting star, and paintbrush. As the Inconsolable Range comes into view, ascend into a rocky basin and pass a shallow, seemingly insignificant pond, which happens to be **lower Chocolate Lake**. Above the lower lake, you cross the stream again and climb up to **middle Chocolate Lake**. ▶5 Campsites spread around a hillside above the north shore will lure overnighters.

Continuing the climb, you switchback up the hillside, cross a willow-lined creek, and reach the **largest of the three Chocolate Lakes**. ▶6 Surrounded by grasses, shrubs, and a few pines, the

Surrounded by grasses, shrubs, and a few pines, the largest of the three Chocolate lakes sits at the base of a talus slope with fine views of the surrounding peaks and ridges.

 Lake

 Camping

 Wildflowers

 Lake

 Camping

Camping

Fishing

lake sits at the base of a talus slope with fine views of the surrounding peaks and ridges. Good campsites spread around the shoreline provide overnight havens for backpackers. All three Chocolate Lakes offer fair fishing for brook trout.

Away from the upper lake, the trail continues its circumnavigation around **Chocolate Peak** on a moderately steep climb across rocky terrain. The USGS 7.5-minute map indicates a pair of trails leading out of the Chocolate Lakes basin and over a ridgecrest to **Ruwau Lake**. Both trails are not maintained well and are a little rough, with sections that virtually disappear for considerable stretches. One path heads directly toward the ridgecrest on a zig-zagging climb up tight switchbacks, while the other path follows longer-legged switchbacks to the crest just southeast of a craggy knob. Whichever way you go, the crest offers fine views of the surrounding terrain. From the ridgecrest, avoid the temptation to directly descend the talus-filled gully below. The two faint paths merge into one and then continue down a hillside above and west of this gully, becoming better defined as you descend. Eventually the north shore of Ruwau Lake is reached. ►7

Lake

Ruwau is perhaps the most scenic of the lakes along the loop, sandwiched between Chocolate Peak and the Inconsolable Range, with fine views from all angles of the neighboring craggy peaks and ridges. On warm afternoons, rock slabs on a tiny island near the north shore will entice swimmers and sunbathers willing to share the chilly, crystalline waters with the resident rainbow trout. Whitebark pines shade campsites on a low hill above the north shore not far from the outlet. Around the remainder of the shoreline, willow thickets and an assortment of wildflowers provide pleasant-looking adornment. Although the lake is only a half mile off the well-traveled Bishop Pass Trail, the area seems just

Wildflowers

far enough off the beaten path to provide an ample helping of solitude and serenity.

The trail heads away from lovely Ruwau Lake toward the outlet and then makes a slight descent through heather and scattered pines. Following a short ascent, the path steeply winds down toward Long Lake and meets the Bishop Pass Trail ►8 at the bottom of the descent.

Turn right and follow gently graded trail through scattered forest and wildflowers past a marshy pond. Soon aptly named **Long Lake** appears through the trees to the left, and **Mt. Goode** cuts a fine profile to the southwest. Farther on, a short climb over a low hump leads directly alongside the picturesque lake. Beyond the far end of the lake, a pronounced descent through thickening forest returns you to the lower junction with the **Chocolate Lakes Trail**. ►9 From there, retrace your steps 1.9 miles to the trailhead. ►10

 Wildflowers

🚶 MILESTONES		
►1	0.0	Start at trailhead
►2	0.75	Straight at Treasure Lakes Trail junction
►3	1.9	Left at lower Chocolate Lakes Trail junction
►4	2.25	Bull Lake
►5	2.8	Middle Chocolate Lake
►6	3.0	Upper Chocolate Lake
►7	3.9	Ruwau Lake
►8	4.5	Right at Bishop Pass junction
►9	5.3	Straight at lower Chocolate Lakes Trail junction
►10	7.2	Return to trailhead

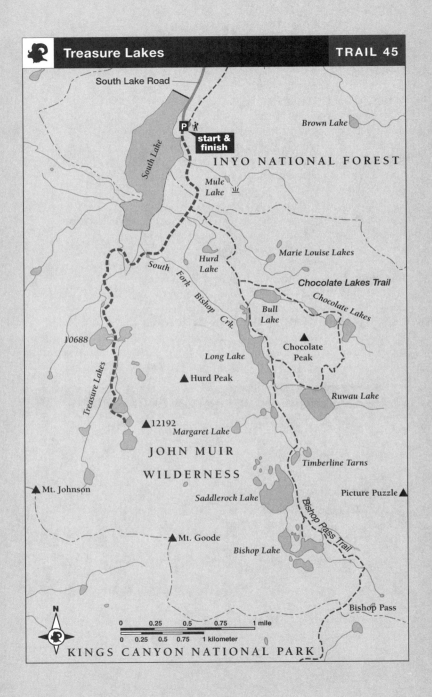

South Lake Road

Brown Lake

P   **start & finish**

INYO NATIONAL FOREST

South Lake

Mule Lake

Marie Louise Lakes

Hurd Lake

South Fork Bishop Crk.

Chocolate Lakes Trail

Chocolate Lakes

Bull Lake

10688

Chocolate Peak

Long Lake

Treasure Lakes

▲ Hurd Peak

Ruwau Lake

▲ 12192

Margaret Lake

JOHN MUIR

WILDERNESS

Timberline Tarns

▲ Mt. Johnson

Saddlerock Lake

Picture Puzzle ▲

Bishop Pass Trail

▲ Mt. Goode

Bishop Lake

Bishop Pass

N

| 0 | 0.25 | 0.5 | 0.75 | 1 mile |
| 0 | 0.25 | 0.5 | 0.75 | 1 kilometer |

KINGS CANYON NATIONAL PARK

Treasure Lakes

While the Bishop Pass Trail may be considered by some to be something of a hikers freeway, the trail branching away toward the Treasure Lakes sees far less traffic. The trail leads to a string of lovely lakes in a secluded granite basin directly below the Sierra Crest. The lakes are quite scenic, offering campers serene surroundings, and providing anglers with excellent fishing for golden trout. Along the relatively short trail, hikers experience three distinct plant zones—montane, subalpine, and alpine. Some route-finding and a bit of boulder-hopping are necessary in order to reach the higher lakes, but travel should be straightforward for most hikers and backpackers. Although equestrians are allowed to use the trail, the absence of a distinct path over rocky terrain discourages horse use above the first two lakes.

Best Time

Snow leaves the area by mid-July, and wildflowers come into season shortly after. By September temperatures have cooled, but the weather is generally favorable until the first storm of the season, usually in late October or early November.

Finding the Trail

Turn west from U.S. Highway 395 in the center of Bishop at Line Drive, and proceed out of town, as the road becomes South Lake Road (Highway 168). Proceed 15 miles to a junction and turn left toward South Lake. Continue another 6.75 miles to the end of the road near the South Lake Dam. Backpackers

TRAIL USE
Dayhike, Backpack,
Run, Horse,
Dogs Allowed

LENGTH
7.6 miles, 3–4 hours

VERTICAL FEET
+1775/-450/±4450

DIFFICULTY
– 1 2 **3** 4 5 +

TRAIL TYPE
Out & Back

FEATURES
Mountain
Lake
Wildflowers
Camping
Swimming
Fishing

FACILITIES
Campground
Resort

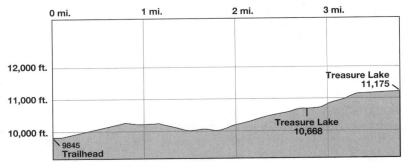

TRAIL 45 Treasure Lakes Elevation Profile

must park in the overnight lot—when this lot is full, additional overnight parking is usually available 1.3 miles back down the road near Parchers Resort (a footpath connects the upper and lower lots). Day-use parking is available just below the overnight lot. Vault toilets and water are available nearby. Four U.S. Forest Service campgrounds are located along South Lake Road: Forks (fee, flush toilets, running water, and phone) Four Jeffrey (fee, flush toilets, and running water), Mountain Glen (vault toilets and fee), and Willow (vault toilets and fee). Resorts strung along South Lake Road include Bishop Creek Lodge, Cardinal Village Resort, and Parchers Resort.

> The trail leads to a string of lovely lakes in a secluded granite basin directly below the Sierra Crest.

Logistics

Backpackers must obtain a wilderness permit for all overnight visits. See page 238 for more details about how to obtain one.

Trail Description

▶1 The well-marked trail begins near the south end of the overnight parking lot, immediately making a very short and steep descent through lush trailside vegetation. A mild climb leads well above the east shore of South Lake through young aspens and lodgepole pines before the trail breaks out into the open to fine views up the canyon of South Fork Bishop Creek. Soon a steeper ascent heads up the hillside past the **John Muir Wilderness boundary** and to a Y-junction with the **Treasure Lakes Trail**. ▶2 Veer right at the junction and head through scattered to light lodgepole pine forest to an easy crossing of a pair of small streams. A mild descent continues, as South Lake pops into view below and Mt. Johnson, Mt. Gilbert, Mt. Thompson, and Hurd Peak appear to the southwest. Proceed to three crossings of South Fork Bishop Creek and two tributaries, where willows, grasses, and wildflowers line the banks. Beyond the third crossing, the real climbing begins in earnest, briefly interrupted by a short descent to the crossing of Treasure Creek.

 Wildflowers

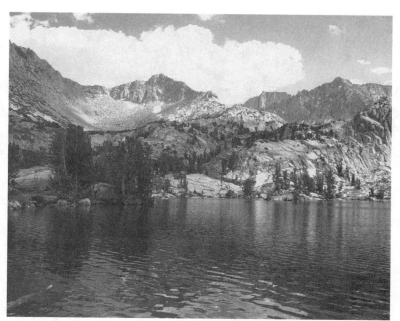

One of the Treasure Lakes

Cross-Country Loop

Rather than retrace your steps back to the trailhead, you could vary your return by following a straightforward off-trail route over a saddle directly south of Peak 12192 and down into the canyon of South Fork Bishop Creek. From the east shore of Lake 11175, climb southeast 550 feet to the prominent saddle and then descend northeast approximately 100 yards before angling over to a tiny creek. Follow the creek briefly and then head straight toward Margaret Lake, where you can pick up a use trail near the northwest shore. Follow the use trail northeast to the south end of Long Lake, ford South Fork Bishop Creek, and shortly meet the Bishop Pass Trail. From there, head generally northwest down the Bishop Pass Trail to the Treasure Lakes Junction and then retrace your steps back to the trailhead.

Continue on a winding, moderately steep ascent beside granite boulders and over granite slabs, and through a mixed forest of lodgepole and whitebark pines. The trail winds back to another crossing of Treasure Creek and continues climbing through a diminishing cover of whitebark pines. Beyond a small pond and a switchback, you arrive at **Lake 10668**, ▶3 the first and largest of the Treasure Lakes. The lake is dotted with small rock islands and bordered by boggy turf along the north shore. A steep wall of rock on the far shore rises up toward **Peak 12047**, providing a fine backdrop to the placid waters. Gently graded tread leads around the east shore, where overnighters will find a number of exposed campsites amid clumps of pine. From the south shore, a use trail branches left to additional campsites near the lake directly east of Lake 10668.

 Lake

 Camping

Continuing south on the main trail, cross a stream and work your way alongside a creek coursing down a rock-filled gully, where clumps of willow and small patches of meadow sprinkled with monkeyflower soften the otherwise stark surroundings.

Where the creek divides into two channels, follow the more gradual cleft on the right through large, blocky talus. Up-canyon, views of Mt. Johnson and the long ridge between it and Mt. Goode add to the rugged alpine scenery. Route-finding from here is straightforward over rocky terrain, as you traverse east to a low ridge and the left-hand fork of the creek, where a **trio of lakes** is cradled in a deep cirque to the west of Peak 12192.

 Mountain

 Lake

The northwest shore of the first of the three lakes has some excellent campsites scattered among whitebark pines. All three lakes should provide anglers with good fishing for golden trout. The route ends at **Lake 11175**. ▶4

 Fishing

🚶	**MILESTONES**		
▶1	0.0	Start at trailhead	
▶2	0.75	Right at Treasure Lakes Trail junction	
▶3	2.8	Lake 10668	
▶4	3.8	Lake 11175	

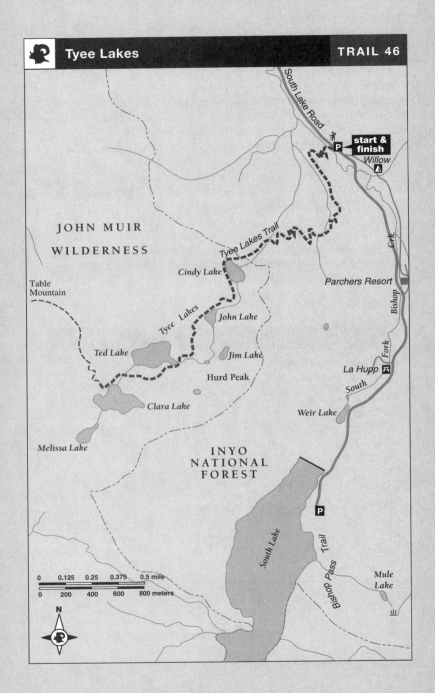

JOHN MUIR

WILDERNESS

Tyee Lakes

The seldom-used Tyee Lakes Trail provides a steep, but short route to a string of delightful lakes set in a high granite basin well east of the Sierra Crest. The 3-mile journey to Clara Lake is well suited for either a dayhike, enhanced by a refreshing swim and a picnic lunch, or an overnight backpack. Thanks to the limited pressure, anglers should find plenty of trout in the Tyee Lakes to keep themselves occupied. A three-quarter-mile, 600-foot climb to a view from the plateau of Table Mountain is a worthy trip extension.

TRAIL USE
Dayhike, Backpack,
Run, Horse,
Dogs Allowed

LENGTH
6.5 miles, 3–4 hours

VERTICAL FEET
+2520/±5040

DIFFICULTY
– 1 2 **3** 4 5 +

TRAIL TYPE
Out & Back

Best Time

The area is snow-free by mid-July, and wildflowers come into season shortly after. By September temperatures have cooled, but the weather is generally favorable until the first storm of the season, usually in late October or early November.

FEATURES
Mountain
Lake
Wildflowers
Camping
Swimming
Fishing

Finding the Trail

FACILITIES
Campground
Resort

Turn west from U.S. Highway 395 in the center of Bishop at Line Drive, and proceed out of town, as the road becomes South Lake Road (Highway 168). Proceed 15 miles to a junction and turn left toward South Lake. Continue another 5.0 miles to the trailhead on the right-hand side of the road and park your vehicle along the gravel shoulder nearby. Four U.S. Forest Service campgrounds are located along South Lake Road: Forks (fee, flush toilets, running water, and phone) Four Jeffrey (fee, flush toilets, and running water), Mountain Glen

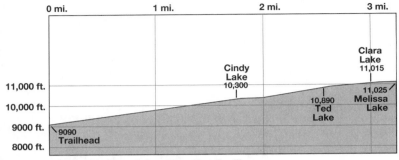

0 mi.	1 mi.	2 mi.	3 mi.

Clara
Lake
11,015

Cindy
Lake
10,300

11,000 ft.

10,000 ft.

11,025
10,890   Melissa
Ted   Lake
Lake

9000 ft.   9090
8000 ft.   Trailhead

TRAIL 46   Tyee Lakes Elevation Profile

(vault toilets and fee), and Willow (vault toilets and fee). Resorts strung along South Lake Road include Bishop Creek Lodge, Cardinal Village Resort, and Parchers Resort.

Logistics

Backpackers must obtain a wilderness permit for all overnight visits. See page 238 for more details about how to obtain one.

Trail Description

▶1 Begin the hike by crossing an impressive, arched, wood bridge over South Fork Bishop Creek. From the far side of the bridge, a moderate, zigzagging climb leads up a sagebrush-covered hillside with pockets of young aspens and lodgepole pines. The steady climb continues, crossing the outlet from Tyee Lakes at 1.5 miles. The grade eases as you enter the **John Muir Wilderness**, round a hill, and approach **Cindy Lake**, passing a pair of fair campsites along the creek on the way to the lakeshore. ▶2 A pleasant beach on the west side invites sunbathers and swimmers, but marshy meadows, clumps of willow, and pockets of aspen border the remaining shoreline. Rising brook trout will surely tempt

 Lake

anglers, although much of the lakeshore is difficult to access due to the dense vegetation.

Arc around Cindy Lake, hop over the trickling inlet dribbling into the lake, and resume the climb. A number of switchbacks lead steeply uphill to grass-rimmed John Lake, the smallest and shallowest of the Tyee Lakes. Across the outlet on top of a granite hump, backpackers will find a few pine-sheltered campsites. Anglers can ply the waters for brook trout.

Leaving the west shore of John Lake, the trail makes a moderately steep climb through whitebark pines over a granite bench. Switchbacks lead to a viewpoint amid dwarf pines and scattered boulders, where you have a bird's-eye vista of **John Lake** below and the tiny lakes to the east of the trail (the largest is Jim Lake). From the viewpoint, a more moderate climb crosses Tyee Creek and passes by a small pond on the way to Ted Lake, ►3 one of the larger Tyee Lakes. Backpackers will find good campsites here sheltered by scattered whitebark pines. An extensive talus slope cascading down the hillside on the far side of the lake provides added scenery.

Skirt the south side of Ted Lake and then begin a moderately steep climb up and over a talus-covered hillside to the narrow cleft holding the stream connecting **Ted Lake** to its upstairs neighbor. Cross this stream and climb up the cleft toward lovely **Clara Lake**, shown as Lake 11015 on the USGS map. ►4 Backdropped by rugged cliffs, Clara is also one of the larger Tyee Lakes, where a few whitebark pines eke out a tentative existence in the near-timberline

Backdropped by rugged cliffs, Clara is also one of the larger Tyee Lakes, where a few whitebark pines eke out a tentative existence in the near-timberline environment.

 Camping

 Lake

Naming the Tyee Lakes

NOTE

Inexplicably, the **Tyee Lakes** were named for a famous brand of salmon eggs. The origin of the various first names applied to each lake (Cindy, John, Jim, Ted, Clara, and Melissa) is unknown.

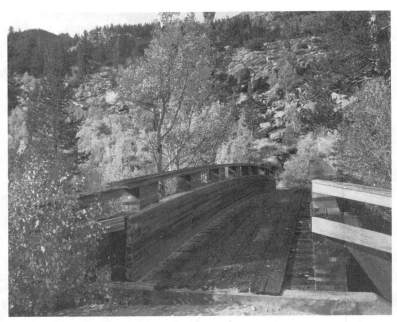

Bridge *over South Fork Bishop Creek, Tyee Lakes Trail*

 Fishing

environment. Unlike at the lower lakes, rainbow trout cohabitate with the characteristic brook trout, which should provide a worthy challenge to any anglers in your group. The last lake in the chain, **Melissa**, ▶5 is a straightforward cross-country jaunt from Clara Lake's southwest shore.

Side Trip to Table Mountain

From Melissa Lake, a 2-mile round-trip to **Table Mountain** will reward you with a dramatic view. Follow a winding climb up the trail through the gorge of a delightful creek that drains into Melissa Lake. Near the head of the gorge, the trail becomes indistinct but the route is obvious—simply head west toward the plateau between Peaks 11684 and 11651, passing through a profusion of corn lilies on the way. With shuttle arrangements, you can continue over Table Mountain and past George Lake (good campsites) to the Lake Sabrina Trailhead.

MILESTONES

▶1	0.0	Start at trailhead
▶2	1.75	Cindy Lake
▶3	2.6	Ted Lake
▶4	3.0	Melissa Lake
▶5	3.25	Clara Lake

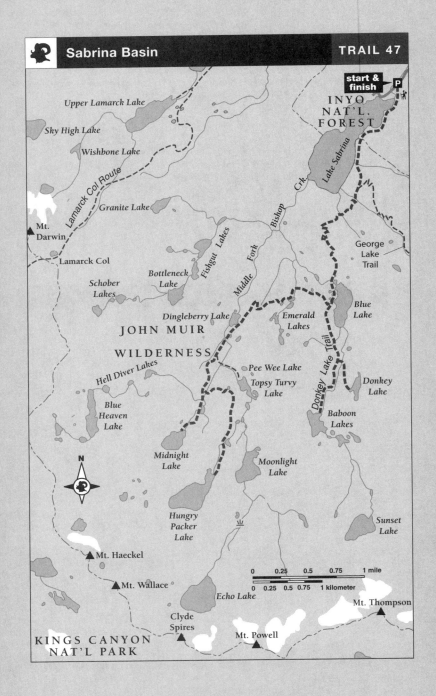

Sabrina Basin

TRAIL 47

start & finish
P

INYO NAT'L. FOREST

Upper Lamarck Lake

Sky High Lake

Wishbone Lake

Lake Sabrina

Lamarck Col Route

Granite Lake

Mt. Darwin

Lamarck Col

Bishop Crk.

George Lake Trail

Fishgut Lakes

Middle Fork

Schober Lakes

Bottleneck Lake

Dingleberry Lake

JOHN MUIR

WILDERNESS

Emerald Lakes

Blue Lake

Donkey Lake Trail

Hell Diver Lakes

Pee Wee Lake

Topsy Turvy Lake

Donkey Lake

Blue Heaven Lake

N

Midnight Lake

Moonlight Lake

Baboon Lakes

Hungry Packer Lake

Sunset Lake

Mt. Haeckel

Mt. Wallace

Echo Lake

Mt. Thompson

Clyde Spires

Mt. Powell

KINGS CANYON NAT'L PARK

0   0.25   0.5   0.75   1 mile
0 0.25 0.5 0.75 1 kilometer

Sabrina Basin

Sabrina Basin holds so many beautiful and worth-while lakes that deciding which ones to visit is often the most challenging part of the trip. With so many lakes to choose from, a healthy dose of solitude and serenity should be fairly easy to get. The lakes of the upper basin are particularly stunning, cradled in granite bowls and encircled by rugged cliffs, with the towering Sierra Crest providing a nearly constant backdrop. Along the way, delightful meadows, colorful wildflowers, cascading streams, and tumbling waterfalls complement the picturesque lakes, while the open nature of the basin offers striking panoramas of the surrounding terrain. Use trails and easy cross-country routes to additional lakes offer plenty of diversions away from the main trail. Whether you're out for just a day, a long weekend, or more, Sabrina Basin has much to offer.

Best Time

Trails are usually snow-free by mid-July, but the lovely meadows of Sabrina Basin reach the height of wildflower season usually from late July through mid-August. Swimmers will find the chilly waters of the lakes the warmest during the month of August. September is a fine time for a visit, although nighttime temperatures may be cold. Snow arrives usually by late October or early November.

Finding the Trail

Turn west from U.S. Highway 395 in the center of Bishop at Line Drive, and proceed out of town, as

TRAIL USE
Dayhike, Backpack,
Run, Horse,
Dogs Allowed
LENGTH
13.6 miles, 7 hours
VERTICAL FEET
+2850/-675/±7050
DIFFICULTY
– 1 2 **3** 4 5 +
TRAIL TYPE
Out & Back

FEATURES
Mountain
Lake
Wildflowers
Camping
Swimming
Fishing

FACILITIES
Campground
Resort

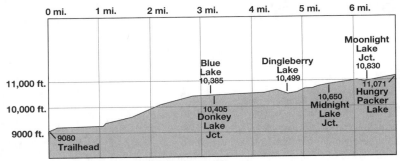

TRAIL 47 Sabrina Basin Elevation Profile

the road becomes South Lake Road (Highway 168). Proceed 15 miles to a junction and continue ahead toward Lake Sabrina, passing the North Lake junction and the overnight parking area (backpackers must park here), to the day-use parking lot near the Lake Sabrina Dam, 3 miles from the South Lake junction. On the way to Lake Sabrina, you pass four U.S. Forest Service campgrounds: Big Trees (fee, flush toilets, and running water), Intake 2 (fee, flush toilets, running water, and bear boxes), Bishop Park (fee, flush toilets, running water, and bear boxes), and Sabrina (fee, flush toilets, running water, bear boxes, and phone). Nearby resorts along South Lake Road include Bishop Creek Lodge, Cardinal Village Resort, and Parchers Resort.

Logistics

Backpackers must obtain a wilderness permit for all overnight visits. See page 238 for more details about how to obtain one.

Trail Description

▶1 Follow the course of an old road away from the day-use parking lot through a cover of aspens until single-track trail leads to a fine vista up the canyon of Middle Fork Bishop Creek. Continue across the open slope, carpeted with sagebrush and dotted with junipers, Jeffrey pines, mountain mahogany, and a few western white pines, above the blue expanse of Lake Sabrina. Toward the far end of the lake, you have a good view of the creek cascading picturesquely into a small cove. Farther up-canyon, the rugged **Sierra Crest** is crowned by the 13,000-foot summits of Mt. Darwin, Mt. Haeckel, Mt. Wallace, and Mt. Powell. Cross into John Muir Wilderness near the lake's midpoint and then begin a steady climb. Reach the junction with the trail to George Lake near the far end of **Lake Sabrina**. ▶2

 Mountain

Immediately cross George Lake's outlet and enter a light forest of lodgepole pines, switchbacking up the slope away from Lake Sabrina and crossing another stream along the way. More switchbacks interspersed with granite steps lead up a hillside, through a rocky ravine, and to a small pond, where the stiff grade abates. Near the pond, the shore of a lake appears through the trees, as you pass a couple of campsites and ford the outlet just below **Blue Lake**. ▶3 The lake is very photogenic,

 Lake

 Lake

Baboon and Donkey Lakes

OPTIONS

A trip to these less visited lakes is a fine way to extend your stay in the area. Head south from the junction near **Blue Lake** through lodgepole pines and around slabs of granite to the crossing of a seasonal stream. From there, a moderate climb leads to an unmarked junction with a faint path heading south-southwest to **Baboon Lakes**. The path disappears before reaching Baboon Lakes, but the route-finding is straightforward alongside the lake's outlet stream to the largest lake. To reach Donkey Lake, continue south from the unmarked junction shortly to the crossing of the creek draining Baboon Lakes, and proceed on faint tread around rock outcrops, past a small pool, and through a notch to the lake. **Donkey Lake** is tucked into a narrow cleft near the base of Thompson Ridge.

Sabrina Basin holds so many beautiful and worthwhile lakes that deciding which ones to visit is often the most challenging part of the trip.

with an irregular shoreline bordered by weather-beaten lodgepole pines and granite benches, and a dramatic backdrop from the craggy, undulating crest of Thompson Ridge. Plenty of campsites are spread around the shoreline, but choose a site wisely, as some are obviously too close to the water to be legal. Anglers can test their skill on brook and rainbow trout. The trail follows the west shore to a three-way junction ►4 with the **Donkey Lake Trail** near the lake's midpoint.

Continuing toward Sabrina Basin, turn right (northwest) from the Donkey Lake junction and follow gently graded trail over a low saddle, across a rocky slope, and then up granite ledges to a grassy vale dotted with lodgepole pines. Cross the outlet from Emerald Lakes and curve around the some-times marshy meadow near the lower lakes to a

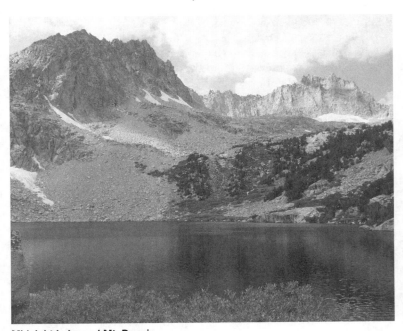

Midnight Lake and Mt. Darwin

Side Trip to Midnight Lake

Scenic Midnight Lake offers an excellent diversion for those with extra time and energy. To reach the lake, veer right at the junction and cross the stream draining Hell Diver Lake. From there, mildly graded trail leads past a fair-size tarn and across the creek draining Midnight Lake to steeper climbing over granite slabs. The grade eases as you crest the lip of a basin and soon stroll over to the north shore of **Midnight Lake**, a teardrop-shaped body of water reposing in a granite bowl surrounded by talus slopes and steep, rugged cliffs. Patches of snow cling to the shady crevices of the cliffs and a waterfall cascades 300 feet into the lake, as 13,831-foot **Mt. Darwin** looms in the background. Near timberline, widely scattered lodgepole pines cling tenuously to cracks in the granite hummocks lining the outlet. While the steep lakeshore inhibits camping, campsites can be found scattered along the creek between the lake and the tarn below.

faint use trail on the left, which provides access to the larger Emerald Lakes. Fine campsites will lure overnighters at the westernmost lake, and anglers should enjoy fishing for brook and rainbow trout. Climb away from Emerald Lakes up granite steps and over granite slabs on the west side of a low ridge and then wind down the far side of the ridge to the southeast shore of **Dingleberry Lake**. ▶5 The lake is squeezed between the cliffs and slabs of a low ridge on one side and the steep wall of Peak 13253's east ridge on the other. Campsites can be found along the creek near both ends of the lake, but the wet meadows on the south end are a haven for mosquitoes in early season.

Beyond the south end of Dingleberry Lake, the foot and stock trails diverge for separate fords of **Middle Fork Bishop Creek**. The two paths reconnect beyond the ford and then climb along a tributary to a picturesque meadow, where the serpentine stream flows lazily through grasses, willows,

 Camping

 Fishing

 Camping

OPTIONS

Moonlight Lake

Austere **Moonlight Lake** is best reached via a use trail below (north of) Sailor Lake, as a vast talus field inhibits access from the main trail to Hungry Packer Lake above. Following the use trail, you ford **Sailor Lake's outlet**, cross a meadow, and then ascend along the outlet from Moonlight Lake to the northwest shore of the rockbound lake. Backpackers will find campsites limited to exposed patches along the outlet and the south end of a low rise above the west shore. In spite of the seemingly lifeless surroundings, the lake hosts a healthy population of brook trout.

Wildflowers

and wildflowers. Across the valley, a dazzling waterfall plunges from **Topsy Turvy Lake**. In the middle of the meadow, a faint use trail heads left toward campsites near Pee Wee and Topsy Turvy lakes. Past the upper end of the meadow, the climb resumes over numerous low granite benches to the Midnight Lake junction. ▶6

From the Midnight Lake junction, head southeast across a pair of willow- and flower-lined creeks, make a mild to moderate climb around a spur ridge. Then head south through scattered whitebark pines to a sloping meadow, filled with willow, heather, and wildflowers sprinkled between glistening granite slabs. A short climb leads to a stunningly picturesque basin brimming with crystalline streams and tumbling cascades, with aptly named Picture Peak in the background. Approximately three-quarters of a mile from the Midnight Lake junction, you reach a junction with a use trail to Moonlight Lake. ▶7

Wildflowers

Great Views

From the Moonlight Lake junction, continue south past **Sailor Lake**, a scenic lake nestled into an open, nearly treeless basin bordered by sloping granite shelves and slabs and pockets of verdant meadow. A number of fine, although exposed, campsites are scattered about the basin, and anglers will find brook and rainbow trout in both the lake and creek.

Proceed up the main trail, with the scenic north face of **Picture Peak** drawing hikers like a scenic beacon. Reach the north shore of **Hungry Packer Lake**, ►8 a narrow finger of water lined by steep cliffs and the towering presence of lovely Picture Peak. During snowmelt, thin ribbons of water cascade majestically down the steep face of the cliffs. A granite peninsula on the northwest shore is too close to the water for legal camping, but the slightly sloping slabs are well suited for afternoon sunbathing. Campsites are limited to a few spots around the outlet. Anglers should find fishing for rainbow trout to be challenging.

▲ Camping

🎣 Fishing

▲ Camping

🚶	**MILESTONES**	
►1	0.0	Start at trailhead
►2	1.25	Straight at George Lake junction
►3	3.2	Blue Lake
►4	3.25	Right at Donkey Lake junction
►5	4.7	Dingleberry Lake
►6	5.5	Straight at Midnight Lake junction
►7	6.25	Straight at Moonlight Lake junction
►8	6.8	Hungry Packer Lake

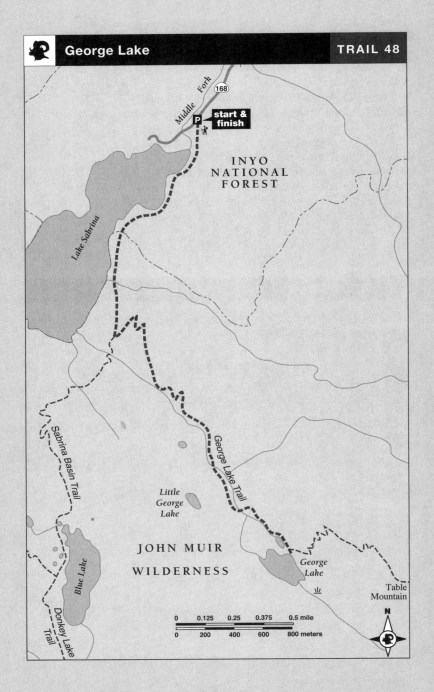

George Lake

TRAIL 48

168

Middle Fork

start & finish

INYO
NATIONAL
FOREST

Lake Sabrina

Sabrina Basin Trail

George Lake Trail

Little
George
Lake

JOHN MUIR

WILDERNESS

Blue Lake

George
Lake

Table
Mountain

Donkey Lake Trail

| 0 | 0.125 | 0.25 | 0.375 | 0.5 mile |

| 0 | 200 | 400 | 600 | 800 meters |

N

George Lake

Although George Lake is not one of the top 10 lakes in Sabrina Basin, it certainly is one of the least crowded, which is something of a mystery, as the delightful lake is only a little over 3 miles from a trailhead. Anglers in search of decent fishing seem to make up the majority of visitors, as backpackers tend to bypass the lake in favor of more distant destinations in Sabrina Basin. Once the anglers head back to the trailhead, campsites at George Lake should offer a considerable amount of peace and quiet. As a backpack or a dayhike, George Lake is a pleasant destination.

Best Time

George Lake is usually snow-free by early July, but the trail over Table Mountain may require another couple of weeks to shed its snow.

Finding the Trail

Turn west from U.S. Highway 395 in the center of Bishop at Line Drive, and proceed out of town, as the road becomes South Lake Road (Highway 168). Proceed 15 miles to a junction and continue ahead toward Lake Sabrina, passing the North Lake junction and the overnight parking area (backpackers must park here), to the day-use parking lot near the Lake Sabrina Dam, 3 miles from the South Lake junction. On the way to Lake Sabrina, you pass four U.S. Forest Service campgrounds: Big Trees (fee, flush toilets, and running water), Intake 2 (fee, flush toilets, running water, and bear boxes), Bishop Park (fee, flush toilets, running water, and bear boxes),

TRAIL USE
Dayhike, Backpack,
Run, Horse,
Dogs Allowed

LENGTH
6.6 miles, 3½ hours

VERTICAL FEET
+1636/-1636

DIFFICULTY
– 1 2 **3** 4 5 +

TRAIL TYPE
Out & Back

FEATURES
Mountain
Lake
Wildflowers
Camping
Swimming

FACILITIES
Campground
Resort

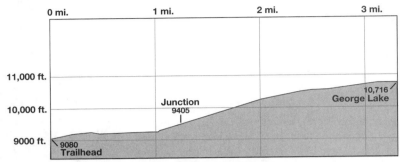

TRAIL 48 George Lake Elevation Profile

and Sabrina (fee, flush toilets, running water, bear boxes, and phone). Nearby resorts along South Lake Road include Bishop Creek Lodge, Cardinal Village Resort, and Parchers Resort.

Logistics

Backpackers must obtain a wilderness permit for all overnight visits. See page 238 for more details about how to obtain one.

Trail Description

▶1 Follow the course of an old road away from the day-use parking lot through a cover of aspens until single-track trail leads to a fine vista up-canyon of Middle Fork Bishop Creek. Continue across the open slope, carpeted with sagebrush and dotted with junipers, Jeffrey pines, mountain mahogany and a few western white pines, above the blue expanse of **Lake Sabrina**. Toward the far end of the lake, you have a good view of the creek cascading picturesquely into a small cove. Farther up-canyon, the rugged **Sierra Crest** is crowned by the 13,000-foot summits of Mt. Darwin, Mt. Haeckel, Mt. Wallace, and Mt. Powell. Cross into the **John Muir Wilderness** near the lake's midpoint and then begin a steady climb. Reach the junction with the trail to George Lake near the far end of Lake Sabrina. ▶2

 Lake

 Mountain

Turn left (northeast) at the junction to follow the **George Lake Trail**, switchbacking moderately steeply up an exposed hillside. Scattered whitebark pines start to dot the slope about a half mile from the junction on the way to a couple of crossings of George Creek. Where the forest cover thickens, near the lower end of a valley, the grade eases and you cross the creek once more near the head of a pleasant-looking meadow. Proceed up the west bank of the creek for a quarter mile, hop over the refreshing brook, and climb above it to circumvent a willow-choked meadow. Another half mile leads to **George Lake**. ▶3

Fine campsites are spread around the north shore of George Lake. Once dayhiking anglers who frequent the lake head back toward the trailhead, backpackers should be able to enjoy a healthy dose of solitude. The hours around sunrise and sunset will usually offer uncrowded fishing for rainbow and brook trout.

As a backpack or a dayhike, George Lake is a pleasant destination.

 Wildflowers

 Lake

 Camping

Shuttle to Tyee Lakes Trailhead

OPTIONS

With a straightforward route over Table Mountain to Tyee Lakes, the 8-mile journey between the **Lake Sabrina and Tyee Lakes trailheads** is an enjoyable 4- to 5-hour hike for advanced hikers. The climb from George Lake to Table Mountain is a worthy out-and-back extension for those with less time. Halfway around George Lake, turn east and follow switchbacks on an increasingly steep grade. The grade eases slightly near the plateau atop **Table Mountain**, and the high point has views of the **Sierra Crest** and surrounding countryside. To continue to South Lake Road, reverse the description for Trail 46 (beginning on page 327).

MILESTONES

▶1   0.0   Start at trailhead
▶2   1.25   Left at George Lake junction
▶3   3.3   George Lake

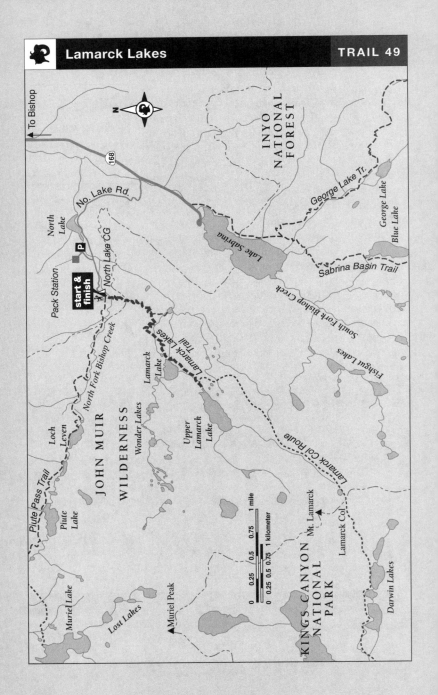

Lamarck Lakes

TRAIL 49

To Bishop

168

INYO NATIONAL FOREST

No. Lake Rd.

North Lake

North Lake CG

George Lake Tr.

George Lake

Blue Lake

Lake Sabrina

Pack Station

P

start & finish

Sabrina Basin Trail

South Fork Bishop Creek

North Fork Bishop Creek

Lamarck Lake

Lamarck Lakes Trail

Fishgut Lakes

Loch Leven

JOHN MUIR WILDERNESS

Wonder Lakes

Upper Lamarck Lake

Lamarck Col Route

Piute Pass Trail

Piute Lake

Muriel Lake

Lost Lakes

Muriel Peak

KINGS CANYON NATIONAL PARK

Mt. Lamarck

Lamarck Col

Darwin Lakes

0   0.25   0.5   0.75   1 mile

0   0.25 0.5 0.75 1 kilometer

Lamarck Lakes

Beautiful lakes and rugged mountain scenery lure hikers and backpackers up the Lamarck Lakes Trail. Although the distance is short, the elevation gain is fairly significant, requiring that visitors be in reasonable condition. Maintained trail dead-ends at Upper Lamarck Lake, which may help to explain the relatively light use the trail receives, but off-trail options to the delightful Wonder Lakes and view-packed Lamarck Col offer fine diversions for those with extra time and energy.

TRAIL USE
Dayhike, Backpack, Run, Horse, Dogs Allowed
LENGTH
5.4 miles, 3 hours
VERTICAL FEET
+1700/-50/±3500
DIFFICULTY
– 1 2 3 **4** 5 +
TRAIL TYPE
Out & Back

FEATURES
Mountain
Lake
Wildflowers
Camping
Swimming
Fishing

FACILITIES
Campground
Pack Station

Best Time

Situated in the rain shadow east of the Sierra Crest, the Lamarck Lakes can be visited as early as the first part of July in years following an average snowfall. Experienced off-trail hikers planning to continue toward Lamarck Col should wait until late July for a mostly snow-free journey. Pleasant weather usually persists in this area through September, with the first snowfall occurring by late October or early November.

Finding the Trail

Turn west from U.S. Highway 395 in the center of Bishop at Line Drive, and proceed out of town, as the road becomes South Lake Road (Highway 168). Proceed 15 miles to the South Lake junction, and continue ahead toward Lake Sabrina 3 miles to the North Lake junction. Turn right and follow the single-lane, gravel road 1.0 mile to the day-use parking area, or 1.6 miles to the right-hand turn into the overnight parking lot directly west of North Lake.

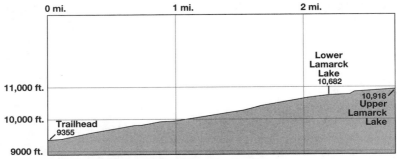

TRAIL 49 Lamarck Lakes Elevation Profile

Both dayhikers and backpackers can be dropped at the trailhead inside North Lake Campground (fee, vault toilets, running water, and bear boxes), but drivers will have to walk the continuation of the North Lake Road from either the day-use or overnight lots to the trailhead. Nearby resorts along South Lake Road include Bishop Creek Lodge, Cardinal Village Resort, and Parchers Resort.

> Lower Lamarck Lake is quite scenic, cradled beneath steep granite cliffs and backdropped by the triangular summit of Peak 12153.

Logistics

Backpackers must obtain a wilderness permit for all overnight visits. See page 238 for more details about how to obtain one.

Trail Description

▶1 From the trailhead inside **North Lake Campground** (1.0 mile from the day-use parking lot and 0.7 mile from the overnight lot), follow single-track trail through aspens and pines a short distance to a junction ▶2 near the edge of the campground.

Veer left at the junction and cross a trio of willow-lined branches of **North Fork Bishop Creek** on wood plank bridges. Past the last bridge, the grade increases to a moderately steep, switch-

backing climb through aspens and lodgepole pines.
Limber pines join the forest on the way to a junction ▶3 with a short path on the left to **Grass Lake**,
which becomes more meadow than lake as the
season progresses.

Veer right at the junction and continue climbing toward Lamarck Lakes through pine forest.
Switchbacks resume where the trail becomes steep,
rocky, and exposed near some cliffs, from where
you have down-canyon views of Grass and North
lakes. Leaving the views behind, the trail heads
back into light forest and continues climbing via
another set of switchbacks. Pass above a small pond
on the right and soon spy the waters of the lower
lake through the trees ahead. A short drop leads to a
crossing of the outlet just below picturesque **Lower
Lamarck Lake.** ▶4

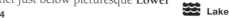 Lake

Lower Lamarck Lake is quite scenic, cradled
beneath steep granite cliffs and backdropped by the
triangular summit of Peak 12153. Clumps of limber

 Mountain

OPTIONS

Wonder Lakes

From Lower Lamarck Lake, a cross-country foray along the outlet
stream to the **Wonder Lakes** is a straightforward enterprise. The
lakes were so named after a packer was sent to plant fish in the
1930s. After some difficulty getting his stock to the lakes, he mar-
veled that he had gotten the job done.

From the northwest shore of **Lower Lamarck Lake**, a steep
climb leads out of the basin, where a use trail can be followed on
the left-hand side of the outlet over rock slabs to the first lake.
Flower-filled meadows, scattered pockets of pines, and numerous
granite slabs border the lakes. Steep cliffs and glacial moraines add
a decidedly alpine character to the surroundings. Less-developed
campsites around the lower lakes provide a more secluded alternative to the overused sites around Lower Lamarck Lake. Anglers can
fish for small brook trout in the lower lakes.

OPTIONS

Cross-Country Route to Lamarck Col

A boot-beaten path has been created over the years almost all the way from the vicinity of Upper Lamarck Lake to 12,920-foot **Lamarck Col** at the Sierra Crest. The high-elevation route is physically demanding, gaining an additional 2800 feet in 2.6 miles, but the high alpine scenery is a just reward. Experienced backpackers use the route over the col as a shortcut to Evolution Basin. To head toward the col, backtrack from Upper Lamarck Lake several hundred yards down the trail, cross Lamarck Creek, and make a short climb southeast on a use trail. Continue past some campsites and a small pond to a sloping meadow bisected by a gurgling stream. Follow ducks on a winding climb alongside this stream to a crossing and then continue the serpentine ascent beside boulders and rocks up a steep hillside. Reach the crest of a ridge, with good views of Grass Lake, Lamarck Lakes, North Lake, Lake Sabrina, and a section of Owens Valley and the White Mountains beyond.

The grade eases for a while on the way around the left side of the ridge through widely scattered pines and spring-fed meadows. From there, the path zigzags more steeply up an arid hillside, followed by an ascending traverse to the base of a steep hill. After surmounting the hill, the route leads into a sloping valley below the Sierra Crest. Climb up this valley toward the perennial snowfield just below the col. Depending on conditions, ascending the snowfield to the col may be difficult. The lofty aerie of Lamarck Col provides a stunning view of Mt. Mendel, Mt. Darwin, and the Darwin Glacier, as well as Darwin Lakes, Darwin Bench, and the deep cleft of Evolution Valley below.

Fishing

pine shade several overused campsites near the outlet and slightly less-used sites above the northeast shore. Fishing in the chilly waters is reported to be fair for rainbow and brook trout.

From Lower Lamarck Lake, the trail proceeds up the rocky wash of **Lamarck Creek**, switchbacking a few times before crossing to the northwest bank. Continue alongside the creek past tiny meadows dotted with pines to the east shore of **Upper**

Lamarck Lake. ►5 The lake, faintly reminiscent of a Norwegian fjord, is tucked into a narrow, steep-walled cirque. The starkness of the environment makes the area seem less hospitable than its lower counterpart. The only break in the cliffs and talus slopes surrounding the lake is found near some stunted pines clinging desperately to a pocket of shallow soil on a rise above the southeast shore. Fine campsites are on this rise and also near some small tarns east of the lake. The upper lake harbors brook and rainbow trout.

 Lake

 Camping

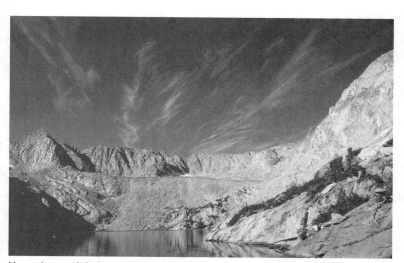

Upper Lamarck Lake

🚶	**MILESTONES**	
►1	0.0	Start at trailhead
►2	0.05	Left at junction
►3	1.0	Right at Grass Lake junction
►4	2.2	Lower Lamarck Lake
►5	2.7	Upper Lamarck Lake

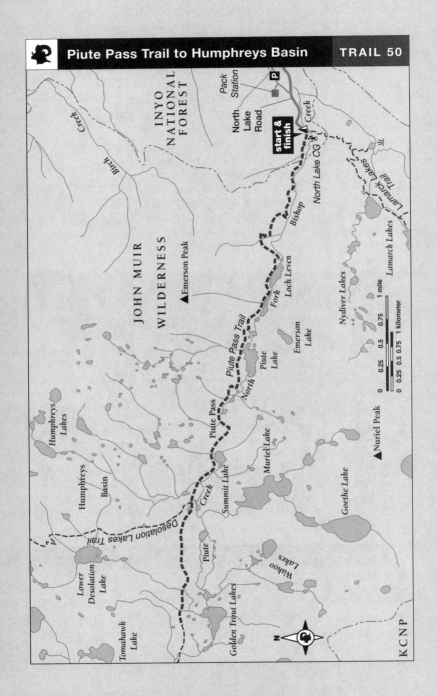

INYO NATIONAL FOREST

Pack Station

P

North Lake Road

Creek

start & finish

North Lake CG

Bishop

Creek

Lamarck Trail

Lamarck Lakes

Birch

Creek

JOHN MUIR WILDERNESS

▲Emerson Peak

Fork

Loch Leven

Piute Pass Trail

Emerson Lake

Nydiver Lakes

North

Piute Lake

1 mile

0.25   0.5   0.75   1 kilometer

0   0.25 0.5 0.75 1 kilometer

Piute Pass

Muriel Lake

▲Nuriel Peak

Humphreys Lakes

Creek

Summit Lake

Goethe Lake

Humphreys Basin

Desolation Lakes Trail

Piute

Wahoo Lakes

Lower Desolation Lake

Golden Trout Lakes

Tomahawk Lake

N

KCNP

Piute Pass Trail to Humphreys Basin

Just north of Glacier Divide, which forms the northern boundary of Kings Canyon National Park, resides a large lake-dotted basin that rivals any in the High Sierra for sweeping alpine beauty. Although much effort is required for the 4.6-mile climb from North Lake (9255 feet) to Piute Pass (11,423 feet), the stupendous scenery abounding in Humphreys Basin is more than an adequate reward. Beyond the pass, gently descending tread leads into the open basin, which has so many worthwhile lakes and tarns for those with rudimentary off-trail skills to visit that deciding where to go may be the hardest part of the whole trip. The lake-dotted basin is rimmed with dramatic peaks and unparalleled alpine scenery that even the most jaded traveler will enjoy.

Best Time

With elevations higher than 11,000 feet, the Piute Pass Trail usually remains snowbound until the middle of July. The wildflower display in Humphreys Basin peaks from late July into early August. September can be a fine time for a hike but be prepared for cold nighttime temperatures as the month progresses. The first significant snowfall usually arrives by late October or early November.

Finding the Trail

Turn west from U.S. Highway 395 in the center of Bishop at Line Drive, and proceed out of town, as the road becomes South Lake Road (Highway

TRAIL USE
Dayhike, Backpack,
Run, Horse,
Dogs Allowed

LENGTH
14.4 miles, 8 hours

VERTICAL FEET
+2175/-650/±5650

DIFFICULTY
− 1 2 3 **4** 5 +

TRAIL TYPE
Out & Back

FEATURES
Mountain
Lake
Wildflowers
Camping
Swimming
Fishing

FACILITIES
Campground
Pack Station

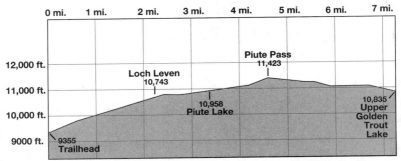

TRAIL 50   Piute Pass Trail to Humphreys Basin Elevation Profile

168). Proceed 15 miles to the South Lake junction, and continue ahead toward Lake Sabrina 3 miles to the North Lake junction. Turn right and follow the single-lane, gravel road 1.0 mile to the day-use parking area, or 1.6 miles to the right-hand turn into the overnight parking lot directly west of North Lake. Both dayhikers and backpackers can be dropped at the trailhead inside North Lake Campground (fee, vault toilets, running water, and bear boxes), but drivers will have to walk the continuation of the North Lake Road from either the day-use or overnight lots to the trailhead. Nearby resorts along South Lake Road include Bishop Creek Lodge, Cardinal Village Resort, and Parchers Resort.

Logistics

Backpackers must obtain a wilderness permit for all overnight visits. See page 238 for more details about how to obtain one.

Trail Description

►1 From the trailhead inside **North Lake Campground** (1.0 mile from the day-use parking lot and 0.7 mile from the overnight lot), follow single-track trail through aspens and pines a short

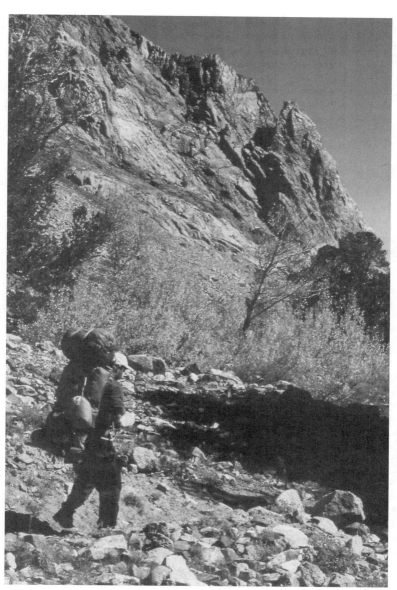

On the Piute Pass Trail

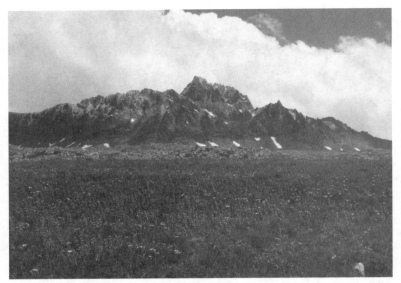

Mt. Humphreys *from Humphreys Basin*

distance to a junction ▶2 near the edge of the campground.

Veer right on the Piute Pass Trail, soon entering the **John Muir Wilderness**, and climb gently through aspen groves, stands of lodgepole pines, and patches of flower-sprinkled meadows. Beyond a pair of log crossings of **North Fork Bishop Creek**, the grade increases to moderate, and the trail ascends away from the canyon floor via a series of switchbacks to a long, ascending traverse. Along the way are excellent views of a waterfall, where the waters of the North Fork plunge steeply from the basin above, as well as Peak 12961 on the left and Mt. Emerson and the multihued Piute Crags on the right. Rock steps and more switchbacks lead up the canyon through diminishing amounts of lodgepole pines and then limber pines. The moderate climb eventually leads you to **Loch Leven**, ▶3 with delightful picnic spots and a few campsites spread

Wildflowers

Lake

Camping

around the lakeshore. Anglers should find fair fishing for brook and rainbow trout.

Leaving the lovely Loch Leven behind, the trail climbs moderately for a short time through scattered lodgepole and whitebark pines to where the grade briefly eases near some ponds. More climbing leads into the next basin and the northeast shore of **Piute Lake**. ►4 Verdant meadows, patches of willow, and widely scattered stands of whitebark pine ring the lake, which is at nearly 11,000 feet, and anglers can test their skill on the resident brook and rainbow trout. Campsites near the trail at Piute Lake are badly overused; backpackers are encouraged to look for spots farther around the wind-prone lakeshore. More remote campsites can be found by scrambling 0.3 mile southeast up a steep slope to rockbound **Emerson Lake**.

From Piute Lake, follow the trail northwest toward timberline, ascending over granite slabs and passing through small meadows sliced by refreshing brooks and dotted with tiny ponds. A final ascending traverse leads to 11,423-foot **Piute Pass**, ►5 where a stunning view of lands both near and far is the reward for all the climbing. Immediately below and west of the pass is the broad expanse of Humphreys Basin, towered over by numerous peaks, including the rugged crest of the Glacier Divide, Muriel Peak, Mt. Goethe, and the nearly 14,000-foot summit of Mt. Humphreys to the north. To the west lie Pilot Peak and the deep cleft of South Fork San Joaquin River. If you're tuckered out from all the high-altitude climbing, Piute Pass makes a fine turnaround point.

Adventurous souls can proceed toward **Humphreys Basin** and a plethora of worthy destinations, where campsites are virtually unlimited, at least for those who don't mind leaving the security of a maintained trail. (Other than a ban within 500 feet of Lower Golden Trout Lake, camping

 Lake

 Fishing

 Camping

 Great Views

is available near any of the numerous lakes and unnamed tarns.) Follow a winding descent around hummocks of granite and past tiny brooks coursing through scenic meadows on long-legged switchbacks well above Summit Lake, where interested anglers may find brook trout gliding through the pale blue waters. Continue the gently graded descent through acres and acres of wildflowers through midseason to a crossing of the outlet from Humphreys Lakes. Here, a faint use trail climbs alongside the stream toward secluded terrain around **Marmot and Humphreys lakes**.

 Wildflowers

A short distance farther is a junction with the distinct but unmaintained trail to massive and austere **Desolation Lake**. Continue down the trail to a faint use trail that heads southwest a relatively short distance to **Upper Golden Trout Lake**, where a number of scenic campsites ring the shore. ►6 The use trail may be hard to locate for first timers, but cross-country travel over open terrain to the lake is straightforward. The massive hulk of nearly 14,000-foot **Mt. Humphreys** above the east edge of the basin dominates the landscape from just about any vantage point.

 Camping

 Mountain

🚶	**MILESTONES**	
►1	0.0	Start at trailhead
►2	0.05	Right at junction
►3	2.2	Loch Leven
►4	3.3	Piute Lake
►5	4.6	Piute Pass
►6	7.2	Upper Golden Trout Lake

Appendix 1

Top Rated Trails

Chapter 1: West Sequoia

3. Eagle Lake
8. Congress Trail
11. Heather, Aster, Emerald, and Pear Lakes
12. Tokopah Falls

Chapter 2: West Kings Canyon

16. Redwood Mountain Grove
22. Lookout Peak
26. Mist Falls

Chapter 3: Golden Trout Wilderness, John Muir Wilderness, and East Sequoia

31. Cottonwood Lakes
33. Mount Whitney

Chapter 4: John Muir Wilderness and East Kings Canyon

40. Brainerd Lake
41. Big Pine Lakes
43. Dusy Basin

Appendix 2

Campgrounds and RV Parks

Campgrounds in the immediate vicinity of trailheads in this guide are listed below, appearing roughly in the same order as the trail descriptions (west side and then east side, south to north). Campgrounds within the national parks are mentioned first, followed by Giant Sequoia National Monument, and then a section of Inyo National Forest campgrounds, which also includes some BLM, county, and privately operated campgrounds. Reservations for National Park Service and U.S. Forest Service campgrounds that accept reservations can be made online at www.recreation.gov, or by calling (877) 444-6777.

Sequoia and Kings Canyon National Parks

South Fork and Mineral King
- South Fork
- Atwell Mill
- Cold Springs

Foothills
- Potwisha
- Buckeye

Generals Highway
- Lodgepole
- Dorst Creek

Grant Grove
- Azalea
- Crystal Springs
- Sunset

Cedar Grove
- Sentinel
- Sheep Creek
- Canyon View
- Canyon View Group
- Moraine

Giant Sequoia National Monument Campgrounds

Generals Highway
Stony Creek
Cove Group
Upper Stony Creek
Fir Group

Big Meadows Area
Buck Rock
Big Meadows

Hume Lake Area
Tenmile
Landslide
Logger Flat Group
Aspen Hollow Group
Hume Lake
Princess

Inyo National Forest Campgrounds

Lone Pine Area
Diaz Lake (Inyo County)
Portagee Joe (Inyo County)
Tuttle Creek (BLM)

Horseshoe Meadow Road
Cottonwood Pass Walk-In
Horseshoe Meadow
Cottonwood Walk-In

Whitney Portal Road
Lone Pine
Lone Pine Group
Whitney Portal
Whitney Portal Group
Whitney Trailhead Walk-In

Independence
Independence Creek (Inyo County)

Onion Valley Road
Lower Grays Meadow
Upper Grays Meadow
Onion Valley

North Oak Creek Drive
Oak Creek

Independence to Big Pine
Goodale Creek (BLM)
Taboose Creek (Inyo County)
Tinemaha (Inyo County)
Baker Creek (Inyo County)
Glacier View (Inyo County)

Glacier Lodge Road
Sage Flat
Upper Sage Flat
Big Pine Creek
Palisade Glacier and Clyde
    Glacier Group Camp

Baker Creek Road

Baker Creek

South Lake Road

Forks
Four Jeffrey
Creekside RV Park (privately
    operated)
Mountain Glen
Willow

Highway 168

Big Trees
Intake 2 Walk-In
Intake 2 Upper
Bishop Park Group
Table Mountain Group
Sabrina

North Lake Road

North Lake

Bishop

Brown's Town
    (privately operated)
Brown's Millpond
    (privately operated)
Horton Creek (BLM)
Highlands RV Park
    (privately operated)
Pleasant Valley (Inyo County)

Appendix 3

Hotels, Lodges, Motels, and Resorts

National Parks

(866) 875-8456, www.nationalparkreservations.com

Sequoia National Park

Wuksachi Lodge

Kings Canyon National Park

Grant Grove Cabins
John Muir Lodge
Cedar Grove Lodge

Giant Sequoia National Monument

Hume Lake Christian Camps, (559) 335-2000, extension 212,
www.humelake.org
Kings Canyon Lodge, (559) 335-2405
Montecito Lake Resort, (800) 227-9900, www.montecitosequoia.com
Stony Creek Lodge, (866) 522-6966,
www.nationalparkreservations.com

Private (Outside the Parks)

Three Rivers

Western Holiday Lodge, (888) 523-9291, www.magnusonhotels.com/
western-holiday-lodge-three-rivers

Buckeye Tree Lodge, (559) 561-5900, www.buckeyetreelodge.com

Comfort Inn and Suites Sequoia Kings Canyon, (559) 561-9010,
www.comfortinn.com

Cort Cottage Bed and Breakfast, (559) 561-4671,
www.cortcottage.com

Gateway Restaurant and Lodge, (559) 561-4133,
www.gateway-sequoia.com

Holiday Inn Express, (800) 315-2621, www.hiexpress.com

Lake Elowin Resort, (559) 561-3460, www.lake-elowin.com

Lazy J Ranch Motel, (559) 561-4449, www.bvilazyj.com

The River Inn, (800) 793-7309, www.the-riverinn.com

Sequoia House, (800) 793-7309, www.sequoiahouse.com

Sequoia Motel, (559) 561-1625, www.sequoiamotel.com

Sequoia River Dance B & B, (559) 561-4411,
www.sequoiariverdance.com

Sequoia Village Inn, (559) 561-3652, www.sequoiavillageinn.com

Sierra Lodge, (888) 575-2555, www.sierra-lodge.com

Three Rivers Motel, (559) 561-4413

Mineral King Road

Silver City Resort, (559) 561-3223, www.silvercityresort.com

Ranch Champagne Cabins, (559) 561-3490,
www.ranchchampagne.com

Appendix 4

Major Organizations

Sequoia Natural History Association

HCR 89, Box 10
Three Rivers, CA 93271
Phone: (559) 565-3759
Fax: (559) 565-3728
www.sequoiahistory.org

The Sequoia Fund

P.O. Box 3047
Visalia, CA 93278
Phone: (559) 739-1668
Fax: (559) 739-1680

National Park Foundation

1201 Eye Street, NW, Suite 550B
Washington, DC 20005
Phone: (202) 354-6460
Fax: (202) 371-2066
www.nationalparks.org

Appendix 5

Useful Books

Backpacking

Beffort, Brian. *Joy of Backpacking*. Berkeley, CA: Wilderness Press, 2007.

Fletcher, Colin, and Chip Rawlins. *The Complete Walker IV*. New York, NY: Knopf, 2002.

O'Bannon, Allen, and Mike Clelland. *Allen and Mike's Really Cool Backpackin' Book: Traveling and Camping Skills for a Wilderness Environment*. Guilford, CT: Falcon Press, 2001.

Guidebooks

Arnot, Phil. *High Sierra, John Muir's Range of Light*. San Carlos, CA: Wild World Publishing/Terra, 1996.

Backpacking California: Mountain, Foothill, Coastal, and Desert Adventures in the Golden State. Berkeley, CA: Wilderness Press, 2008.

Jenkins, J. C., and Ruby Johnson Jenkins. *Exploring the Southern Sierra: East Side*. Berkeley, CA: Wilderness Press, 1992.

———. *Exploring the Southern Sierra: West Side*. Berkeley, CA: Wilderness Press, 1995.

Krist, John. *50 Best Short Hikes in Yosemite and Sequoia/Kings Canyon*. Berkeley, CA: Wilderness Press, 1993.

Morey, Kathy. *Hot Showers, Soft Beds, and Dayhikes in the Sierra: Walks and Strolls Near Lodgings*. 3rd ed. Berkeley, CA: Wilderness Press, 2008.

Morey, Kathy, Mike White, et al. *Sierra South. Backcountry Trips in California's Sierra Nevada*. 8th ed. Berkeley, CA: Wilderness Press, 2006.

Roper, Steve. *Climbers Guide to the High Sierra*. San Francisco: Sierra Club Books, 1995.

————. *Sierra High Route: Traversing Timberline Country.* Seattle: The Mountaineers Books, 1997.

Schaffer, Jeffrey P., Ben Schifrin, et al. *Pacific Crest Trail: Southern California.* 6th ed. Berkeley, CA: Wilderness Press, 2003.

Secor, R. J. *The High Sierra, Peaks, Passes, and Trails.* 2nd ed. Seattle: The Mountaineers Books, 1999.

Sorensen, Steve. *Day Hiking Sequoia: Fifty Day Hikes for Sequoia National Park.* 2nd ed. Three Rivers, CA: Fuyu Press, 1996.

Spring, Vicky. *100 Hikes in California's Central Sierra and Coast Range.* 2nd ed. Seattle: The Mountaineers Books, 2004.

Stone, Robert. *Day Hikes in Sequoia and Kings Canyon National Parks.* 2nd ed. Red Lodge, MT: Day Hike Books, Inc., 2001.

White, Mike. *Kings Canyon National Park: A Complete Hiker's Guide.* Berkeley, CA: Wilderness Press, 2004.

————. *Sequoia National Park: A Complete Hiker's Guide.* Berkeley, CA: Wilderness Press, 2004.

History and Literature

Browning, Peter. *Place Names of the Sierra Nevada.* Berkeley, CA: Wilderness Press, 1991.

Dilslayer, Larry M., and William C. Tweed. *Challenge of the Big Trees.* Three Rivers, CA: Sequoia Natural History Association, 1990.

Farquahar, Francis P. *History of the Sierra Nevada.* Berkeley, CA: University of California Press, 1965.

Jackson, Louise A. Buelah. *A Biography of the Mineral King Valley of California.* Tucson, AZ: Westernlore Press, 1988.

Strong, Douglas H. *From Pioneers to Preservationists: A Brief History of Sequoia and Kings Canyon National Parks.* Three Rivers, CA: Sequoia Natural History Association, 2000.

Tweed, William. *Beneath the Giants: A Guide to the Moro Rock-Crescent Meadow Road of Sequoia National Park.* Three Rivers, CA: Sequoia Natural History Association, 1986.

————. *Kaweah Remembered.* Three Rivers, CA: Sequoia Natural History Association, 1986.

Natural History

Cutter, Ralph. *Sierra Trout Guide.* Portland, OR: Frank Amato Publications, 1991.

Horn, Elizabeth L. *Sierra Nevada Wildflowers.* Missoula, MT: Mountain Press, 1998.

Johnston, Verna R. *Sierra Nevada: The Naturalist's Companion.* Rev. ed. Berkeley, CA: University of California Press, 1998.

Laws, John Muir. *The Laws Field Guide to the Sierra Nevada.* Berkeley, CA: Heyday Books, 2007.

Moore, James G. *Exploring the Highest Sierra.* Stanford, CA: Stanford University Press, 2000.

Petrides, George A., and Olivia Petrides. *Western Trees.* New York: Houghton Mifflin, 1998.

Smith, Genny, ed. *Sierra East: Edge of the Great Basin.* Berkeley, CA: University of California Press, 2000.

Weeden, Norman F. *A Sierra Nevada Flora.* 4th ed. Berkeley, CA: Wilderness Press, 1996.

Whitney, Stephen. *A Sierra Club Naturalist's Guide.* San Francisco: Sierra Club Books, 1979.

Index

Author

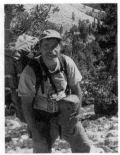

Mike White

Mike White was raised in the suburbs of Portland, Oregon, in the shadow of Mt. Hood (whenever the Pacific Northwest skies cleared enough to allow such things as shadows). As a teenager, Mike began hiking, backpacking, and climbing in the Cascades of Oregon and Washington and then honed his outdoor skills while attending Seattle Pacific University.

After acquiring a B.A. in political science, Mike and his new wife, Robin, relocated to Reno, Nevada. In the early 1990s, Mike left his last "real" job (with an engineering firm), and began writing full time. His first project for Wilderness Press was an update and expansion of Luther Linkhart's classic guide, *The Trinity Alps*. His first solo project was *Nevada Wilderness Areas and Great Basin National Park*. He is the author of the popular Snowshoe series, as well as guides to Lassen Volcanic, Kings Canyon, and Sequoia national parks, as well as guides to the Reno-Tahoe area. Mike has contributed to *Backpacking California, Sierra North*, and *Sierra South* and has written for *Sunset* and *Backpacker* magazines, as well as the *Reno-Gazette Journal*.

Mike teaches hiking, backpacking, and snowshoeing classes at a local community college and dispenses trail information while working part time at REI. He lives in Reno with his wife, Robin, and their youngest son, Stephen, along with their two labs. David, Mike and Robin's oldest son, still resides in the area with his wife, Candace.

Series Creator

Joe Walowski

Joe Walowski conceived of the Top Trails series in 2003, and was series editor of the first three titles: *Top Trails Los Angeles, Top Trails San Francisco Bay Area*, and *Top Trails Lake Tahoe*. He currently lives in Seattle.